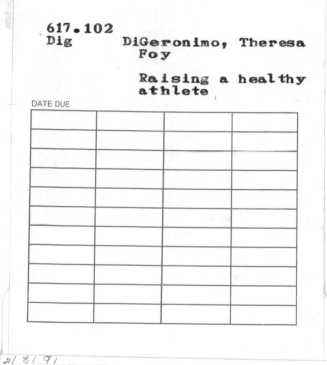

617.102
Dig   DiGeronimo, Theresa
             Foy

             Raising a healthy
             athlete

DATE DUE

2/ 8/ 9/

Raising a Healthy Athlete

RAISING A HEALTHY ATHLETE

Douglas G. Avella, M.D.
and
Theresa Foy DiGeronimo, M.Ed.

British American Publishing

Illustrations by Ken Morris, Jr., MA., A.M.I.

Library of Congress Cataloging-in-Publication Data

DiGeronimo, Theresa Foy.
  Raising a healthy athlete / Theresa Foy DiGeronimo &
Douglas G. Avella.
    p. cm.
  ISBN 0-945167-36-9 :
  1. Pediatric sports medicine. 2. Sports for children—Health
aspects. I. Avella, Douglas G., 1951-   . II. Title.
RC1218.C45D54   1990
617.1'027—dc20   90-1608
                                                          CIP

Published by British American Publishing
19B British American Boulevard
Latham, NY 12110

Manufactured in the United States of America

94 93 92 91 90 5 4 3 2 1

The ideas, procedures and suggestions contained in this book
are not intended as a substitute for consulting with your
physician. All matters regarding your child's health require
medical supervision.

To my wife, Elizabeth.
And to my two future Olympians, Jillian and Nicholas,
who make every day a new experience.
D.G.A.

To my son, Matt, whose years of sports injuries have
piqued my interest in this field of medicine and whose
fractured wrist put me in touch with Dr. Avella.
T.D.

Contents

Acknowledgments

We would like to acknowledge the help of the following coaches who, by reviewing the chapters in Part II, helped us keep the information in this book accurate and up to date: Jack DeSalvo, baseball; Dan Fehlberg, gymnastics; Dennis Goldman, football; Bill Matarazzo, track and field; Lisa Rademacher, volleyball; Joe Ross, football; Gustav Schell, soccer; Kate Stewart, tennis; Pat Taliaferro, softball.

We would like to add a special word of thanks to Ken Morris, Jr., MA., A.M.I. our illustrator, Terry W. Hensle, M.D., who helped us prepare the chapter about an athlete's diet, and Mike Weis, ATC, who was a constant source of instant information.

I (D.G.A.) would personally like to thank those physicians who most influenced me in the study of orthopedics: Robert Fernand, M.D., and Phillip Cohen, M.D. Also, E. Robert Wilson, M.D., whose devotion to the handicapped child kindled my interest in children's orthopedics, Wallace Lehman, M.D., my mentor at the Hospital for Joint Diseases in New York, and Michael G. Ehrlich, M.D., my pediatric orthopedic preceptor who gave me many hours of devotion, dedication, and hard work during my fellowship at the M. G. H. Also, thank you to Joseph Pizzurro, M.D., for his kindness and generosity, Raymond Reddin, Esq., a tried and true friend, and T.D., my co-author, whose persistence made this book a reality.

ix

Introduction

An estimated 12 to 15 million American children play organized sports each year; several million of these young athletes sustain sports-related injuries. As a pediatric orthopedist, Dr. Avella knows firsthand the risk factors that are inherent in sports play and how this worries parents. Time and time again parents of injured athletes ask him if there is any way they could have prevented the accident and if they should forbid their child to continue playing the sport. Unfortunately, there aren't "correct" answers to these questions, but it is our hope that the information in this book will help clarify your role in the prevention and care of sports injuries and give you the facts you need to establish and monitor safe athletic programs.

The social, psychological, and physical benefits that can be derived from sports activities are innumerable. The long list of positive attributes includes the development of self-esteem, self-discipline, and self-confidence. Your child's involvement in athletics can foster dedication, concentration, cooperation, and acceptance in the peer culture. Young competitors learn to put individual ambition aside to work toward team goals, and they learn about fairness, conflicts, and competition. Also, participation can improve physical health, refine motor skills, and foster a life-long appreciation of personal fitness. All of these, along with the fact that sports play can be just plain fun, explain why parents like you encourage children to be active in athletics despite the fact that all sports present the potential for injury.

Raising a Healthy Athlete will give you the information you need to enhance the positive qualities of sports involvement and reduce the risks. It will also show you why when you hand over your children to the coaches, you do not hand over the primary responsibility for their health and welfare. Experts agree that the more parents know about their role in the sports program, the way growing bodies work, and how injuries can be prevented, the more likely it is that children will have enjoyable and healthy sports experiences.

The information in this book is organized in three parts. Part I explains how you can prevent injuries regardless of the sport your child plays. This is possible because the majority of sports-related injuries are not caused by the sport itself, but by negligent circumstances such as poor supervision, improper use or lack of equipment, and insufficient physical conditioning. These are all risk factors that, very often, you can control. In this section you will read about the importance of monitoring your children's diet and sleep habits so that they perform in optimal physical shape. Then, to enhance physical ability, you can use information in Part I to monitor a conditioning regime that will foster flexibility, agility, speed, cardiovascular endurance, muscular endurance, and muscular strength. You will understand the necessity of pre-season physicals even when they are not required by the sports organization, and you will be instructed how to determine if your child needs a more thorough examination than can be administered at a "team" physical. Finally, Part I alerts you to the dangers of sports participation which include fad diets, anorexia nervosa, bulimia, steroid abuse, and burnout.

Part II examines ways to avoid injury in 14 popular sports. Although it is impossible in this book to offer a comprehensive look at all aspects of these sports, you will find a thorough discussion of specific injury-related factors such as use of equipment, practice sessions, proper technique, causes of common injuries, and suggestions for conditioning the body parts stressed by each sport. This information, combined with the strategies suggested in Part I, will keep you well armed to protect your young athlete from injury.

Part III gives guidelines to help you care for sports injuries. You will learn facts of anatomy that will help you understand the kinds of physical activities most likely to injure the immature musculoskeletal system of young athletes. It also explains why it is dangerous to treat some youth injuries in the same manner recommended for adults; what is appropriate for adult muscles, bones, ligaments, and cardiovascular functioning is not always applicable to your child. This will be followed by an alphabetical listing of common sports-related injuries and an explanation of causes, symptoms, treatment, prevention tips, and rehabilitation information. Emphasis is placed on minor traumas that constitute nearly 95 percent of youth sporting injuries. These include heat exhaustion and stroke, shock, blisters, floor burns, skin irritations, nose bleeds, aching muscles, bruises, muscle pulls, sprains and strains, cuts and abrasions. These facts will support your decision to say "No" when an injured child wants to play when hurt rather than disappoint the team or the coach. They will also help you supervise the rehabilitation process so that your child does not risk the same injury again by returning to active play too soon and yet is not barred from participation longer than necessary. To assure that no child is unnecessarily excluded from sports play, Part III includes a discussion of physical activity for children with chronic illnesses as well as for those with mental or physical handicaps. Sports can be especially beneficial for these athletes when parents, doctors, and coaches recognize and work with their special needs.

This book also recognizes that sports programs are not for boys only. Fifteen years ago, books about youth athletics focused on male athletes because at that time boys dominated the school and community sports programs. Today, however, millions of American girls are also enjoying a full range of athletic activities; in fact, many high schools offer as many as 27 female competitive scholastic sports programs. Obviously, parents need sports-injury information for both their sons *and* their daughters. For this reason *Raising a Healthy Athlete* addresses the needs of the male and female athlete and uses sometimes awkward grammatical constructions to include them both.

Sports play gives boys and girls many positive life skills and attitudes and is wholeheartedly endorsed by The American Academy of Pediatrics. Nothing in this book is intended to scare you or to condemn athletic programs or coaches. Rather, we intend to give you, the parents of young athletes, the knowledge and confidence you need to recognize dangerous situations and take steps to correct them so that preventable injuries do not happen. The book is based on sound medical facts and procedures gathered through Dr. Avella's experience as an athlete and as an orthopedist treating children with sports-related injuries. It is not, however, intended to take the place of your own doctor's advice. Use the suggestions to help prevent sports-related injuries, but if such injuries do occur, use it to evaluate the problem, to determine if your child needs professional medical attention, and to better understand your doctor's prescribed course of treatment. If you use *Raising a Healthy Athlete* in this way, you will find yourself constructively involved in youth athletics and well on your way to assuring your child a safe and enjoyable sports experience.

Part I
Prevention of
Sports Injuries

1

■■■■■

Parents and Coaches and the Foundation of Injury Prevention

When your sons and daughters join sports teams, you deliver them into the hands of coaches who teach them the rules, skills, and strategies of the game. These coaches will decide which position which kids should play, how often they should practice, who should be on the first team, or if the team strategy is to win at all costs. At the practices and games, the coaches are in charge. Even though you, the parent, are not the authority figure in the sports arena, you do not relinquish total control of your child's physical and mental well-being. You *and* the coach become a team that must work together to ensure safe and enjoyable sports participation. Although walking the middle road between stepping aside and remaining involved in your child's athletic programs is sometimes like taking a gallop spring on a balance beam, it is an important factor in protecting your young athlete from sports-related injuries. The information in this chapter will

7

help you define and balance your roles as parent and spectator by clarifying your responsibility in keeping your children healthy.

Certainly, as a parent you already know a great deal about this. You know what to do when your children have fevers or cut elbows, chicken pox or ear infections. But how much do you know about *preventing* sports-related injuries? Test your knowledge by asking yourself what you would do in these situations:

1. When up at bat, your child gets hit in the ribs with a wild pitch. After several seconds of painful squirming in the dirt, he or she is picked up by the coach and pushed to run toward first base.
2. Your 9-year-old has pitched every inning of a baseball game because the alternate pitcher didn't show up for the game. The team is about to go into extra innings and once again your child heads out to the pitcher's mound.
3. Your son rushes out the door anxious to be early for his first high school football practice. This pre-season practice is being "supervised" by the team captain in 90° August heat.
4. Your child has mentioned that the new coach is a real tough drill sergeant. For the last three weeks your young athlete has been suffering from sore muscles, chronic fatigue, and irritability.
5. Your young basketball player is sent home from a practice with a sprained collar bone. The team trainer tells you that he or she will be on the bench for at least two weeks. Two days later the coach calls to tell you that he's talked it over with the trainer, and they feel your child will be able to play in this week's big game.
6. As you watch your child's team play its rival, you hear the coach shout, "Don't come off that field until one of their players comes back in a body bag!"
7. Your football player brings home a helmet that is old,

worn, and several sizes too big. The coach apologizes for the shabby equipment, but explains that there's no more money in the budget to buy new ones.

These kinds of scenarios are played out every day in every town in America. As you were reading them over, you probably knew something was wrong and that, as a parent, you should do something about it. But what? If you were in these situations, do you think you would step in and become involved? Or would you stay out of it and hope that the kids and the coaches know what they're doing?

This "should-I-butt-in" dilemma exists because very often parents aren't sure what's just part of the game and what's really harmful to their kids. They don't want to appear overprotective, yet by ignoring the situation they could risk their child's health. One way to assure that you know how to respond is to learn all you can about the sport your child is playing, the causes of sports-related injuries, and the basics of children's physiology and rehabilitation.

Learning the Facts

The first line of defense in injury prevention is found in the rules of the game: all organized sports have safety regulations. Some coaches and officials carefully follow them and put the well-being of the athlete over the outcome of the game. Others, unfortunately, either lack familiarity with these standards or choose to ignore them. That's why you should learn the rules of the game. When you do, you'll feel confident stepping in to remedy a few of the unhealthy situations cited above. For example:

• To avoid elbow injury, often called Little League elbow, elementary school pitchers are only allowed to pitch three innings per game and they are not allowed to throw curve balls. Therefore, you won't be overstepping your parental boundaries when you ask the coach to give your child's arm a rest, even if that means a less proficient pitcher may have to finish out the game. The safety rules make this an acceptable option.

• You'll also feel comfortable about keeping your son home from unofficial and unsupervised summer football practices if you know that, by league rules, a player is not allowed to work out with the team unless three conditions are met: the player must pass the team physical, an adult must supervise each practice, and the team can not practice before the official starting date.

• Any football player on any organized team at any level of play must be issued a helmet certified each year for safety and quality by the National Operating Committee on Standards for Athletic Equipment (NOCSAE). Knowing this, you're right to insist that the team, the town, the school, the league, or the parents as a group appropriate the funds for proper equipment before the kids step onto the playing field.

With persistence, you'll certainly be able to obtain a copy of the game's rules. First ask the team coach; a good one will be glad to lend you his or her own copy. If the coach doesn't have a handbook of rules, take a trip to your local library and look in both the children's and adults' card catalogs under the name of the specific sport. If that too fails, write to the appropriate organization listed in Appendix B and ask for an official rule book.

The rules of the game are created to promote fairness and safety. Before the season begins, all coaches, parents, and athletes should know what they are.

Next, you'll need some basic information about the young athlete's developing musculoskeletal system. Knowing how the bones, muscles, and ligaments work, grow, and injure will help you decide when your son or daughter can "work through the pain" and when he or she needs medical attention. This information, explained in Chapters Three and Fifteen, will help you recognize the signs of over-training, and understand the necessity for warm-ups, cool-downs, and body conditioning (as explained in Chapter 3). Also, because studies of sports-related accidents consistently find that many injuries are actually *re*-injuries, you'll need to know something about the rehabilitation process. If the coach calls and tells you it's "okay" for your child to play before he or she is fully healed, you'll know how to handle the situation. See Chapter Seventeen for information about the rehabilitation of common sports-related injuries.

Knowledge is your number one weapon in warding off sports injuries before they happen. Be sure to stock up on the facts before you send your child out onto the playing field.

Checking Your Attitude

With a basic understanding of sporting rules and developmental physiology in mind, it's time to examine your own attitudes towards your young athlete's involvement in a sports program. The expectations you set, the philosophies you espouse, and the emphasis you place on winning will all affect your ability to prevent sports-related injuries.

Do You Want Your Child To Play?

If you want your children to play organized sports, it will be easy for you to give them your full support and encouragement. Just make sure that your children want to play as much as you want them to. Kids whose parents push them into sports are more prone to injury for a number of reasons. These children often have an attitude that says, "I don't want to be here, so I'm not going to listen to the rules, or wear my safety equipment, or respect the rights of the other players." They can become a danger to themselves and to others. Pushed children may also be trying to master playing skills for which they are not physically or developmentally ready.

Most kids have good insight into what they can and cannot do. An "I don't want to" response can really mean "I can't." Listen to your children and follow their lead.

If your sons or daughters do not want to play a particular sport, don't make them. Instead, find out what they are interested in doing (be it another sport, music, art, dance, or scouting). If you support their choices, children can attain the same positive experiences and life lessons from other extracurricular activities as they do from sports.

If, after investigating the requirements and injury patterns of a particular sport, you *don't* want your children to play, you have two choices: 1) forbid them to play, or 2) give your permission and keep your misgivings to yourself. Elaine, for example, didn't want her son Ken to go out for football. But Ken had his heart set on playing, and his dad thought it was a good idea. Elaine reluctantly gave her permission but only after making it perfectly clear how much she disapproved. Then, each time Ken went to play, she'd remind him, "You'd better be careful when you play. I'm warning you, football is a dangerous game. I don't want you to get hurt. You know, some kids end up paralyzed because they play this game. Don't you go and get hurt." Poor Ken. When he's out on the field, he worries more about getting hurt than he thinks about what's going on in the game. This worry affects his ability to participate wholeheartedly, and this hesitation makes him *more* prone to injury.

Children who know their parents are waiting to pounce with an "I told you so" at the first sign of trouble are also at increased risk for injury. It is very likely that if Ken gets hurt in a game, he will avoid telling his mother about it. He certainly would rather play in pain or ignore symptoms of body stress than admit that she was right.

If you give your son or daughter permission to play, give it without condition, reservation, or incessant, worried warnings.

Why Do You Want Your Child To Play?

While waiting for the high school girls' basketball game to begin, one father was overheard talking about his daughter. He was explaining to another parent why he wanted her to play the game. "Basketball has been great for Karen," he began. "She really loves the game and it has put her in contact with other girls who share the same interest. This coach has really piqued her interest by teaching proper techniques and exciting game strategies."

If you look closely at this conversation, you'll notice that this father never once used the word, "I." Other parents might have said, "I want my daughter to play basketball because I love to watch her play. I'm proud of her ability. I've told her that if she really tries, I think she has enough talent to be an all-star. I always wanted to be good in basketball, but I didn't have the talent she does."

Karen's father wants his daughter to play this sport because it seems to be good for her, not him. Karen is a lucky athlete. She can go onto the court without feeling parental pressure to perform in a certain way. She doesn't need to push herself beyond her natural capabilities in order to live up to her dad's expectations. And she doesn't need to feel ashamed or like less of a daughter if she has a bad game. In encouraging her to enjoy herself, this dad is protecting his daughter from injuries caused by undue pressure to achieve. You too can prevent injuries by never saying or implying to your athlete, "When you look good, I look good."

What Kind Of A Coach Do You Admire?

Coaches come in all shapes and sizes, and with any number of management techniques and sports philosophies. If you had a choice, which of the following two kinds of coaches would you choose for your 9-year-old child? HAL: Hal makes optimal use of his best players, and explains to the kids left on the bench that winning is a team effort; their contribution is to cheer their team on. This coach barks out commands, holds frequent, demanding, and long practices, and comes up with a winning team every year. Each new year he opens the season with a promise to the kids and to their parents, "We're gonna work hard and we're gonna do whatever we have to do to stay number One!" JACK: Jack plays all the members of the team in equal time periods. At practice he focuses on proper technique, and all players practice all positions. Jack rarely yells; when he sees a problem situation he runs over to the player and talks it over quietly. Unfortunately, Jack's team rarely wins. In fact, they've been last in the league for three years in a row. At the start of this year's season he promised the kids and their parents, "I don't know if we'll be number one, but I do know that we're sure gonna try. I can also promise you that every player will learn how to play, and every player will have a chance to play in every game."

It's easy to see that Jack is the better teacher, but if his team loses, is Hal the better coach? From the standpoint of injury prevention (both physical and mental), Jack wins hands down. The members of his team will learn good technique which will save them from the injuries caused by improper body movement. In practice situations athletes will learn to adjust their skills to different playing positions; this gives less proficient players the chance to play, improve their skills, and safely prepare for the time when they need to replace a first-string teammate who is absent or injured. Such an approach to training will also decrease the rate of drop-out due to boredom. The better players, meanwhile, won't be overworked, which will reduce their risk of fatigue-related injuries.

Surely, there are hundreds of thousands of parents who, deep down inside, want their young athletes to play the same sports they played or dreamed of playing, and they want them to be the stars and to win at any cost. If you feel this way, you're not alone. But if you sincerely seek to protect your children from sports-related injuries and you want them to continue playing sports in the future, put *their* feelings first, and put enjoyment before winning.

This does not mean that you should completely de-emphasize winning. Competing and wanting to win is a part of life and a measure of success in any endeavor. You and your athlete should always strive to win, but not at the cost of physical or mental injury.

You can best demonstrate this attitude through your behavior at sporting events. The National Association for Sport and Physical Education (NASPE) recommends the following standards as an unofficial code of conduct for sports parents:

- Remain seated in the spectator area during the game.
- Don't yell instructions or criticism at the athletes.
- Refrain from making derogatory comments to players or parents of the opposing team, to officials, or to league administrators.
- Do nothing that will detract from the enjoyment your child gets from the sport.

Armed with knowledge of the sport, the basics of sports medicine, and an appropriate attitude, you'll be a more effective monitor of the sports program itself.

Examining Safety Equipment

Every athlete needs the safety equipment appropriate to his or her sport. In Part II of this book, the equipment that is absolutely necessary in a variety of popular youth sports is itemized and discussed. Be sure to read over these lists to make sure that your athlete has the appropriate gear.

Some sporting programs have certified coaches and/or trainers who ensure that each athlete has equipment in good condition that fits properly; unfortunately, the majority of programs do not. Therefore it's up to you to make sure your children are outfitted adequately enough to protect them from injury. Ask your child HOW the equipment was distributed; it should never be handed out on a first-come, first-served basis. It is very unlikely that equipment which is blindly doled out to whomever is next in line will fit properly; it will most likely be either too small or too large.

Schedule a personal equipment inspection at least once in the beginning of the season. If team rules prohibit your child from bringing equipment home, tell the coach why you want to see it. Assure him or her that it will be returned promptly, or offer to go down to the playing field and inspect the equipment there. If you're not sure if the equipment is of sufficient quality or proper fit, you should be able to find a certified trainer at the local high school, college, or hospital who will either tell you over the phone what to check for, or who will be willing to take a look if you bring your child and the equipment in for inspection. The information in Part II of this book will also give you some basic safety criteria to follow when examining safety equipment.

Knowing the Value and Purpose of Practice Sessions

Every aspect of practice sessions plays a role in either preventing or causing sports-related injuries. The practice should always include instruction on proper technique. This is especially so in youth leagues where youngsters are just learning the skills of the game. If, for example, young football players spear opponents with their helmets, or baseball/softball players block the plate to make a tag, or tennis players consistently make late contact with the ball, they open themselves to preventable injuries. Professional players know how to absorb impact, how to hit, throw, run, block, and kick. In short, they use their bodies to complement, rather than work against, the physical demands of the sport. Young players are always in danger of injury until they learn proper technique. Therefore, your young athlete should know that racking up a winning score (which is sometimes more easily done using improper playing technique) is not as important as learning to play correctly.

During practice sessions and throughout the sport season, watch your young athlete for signs of over-training. This happens when an athlete trains at a continually high intensity without giving the body enough rest time to completely or efficiently recover its strength. The symptoms of over-training are discussed in detail in Chapter Three.

At practice sessions you should also watch to see if all players are actively involved. Note if some athletes stand by idly while the "stars" are coached and encouraged. If so, some team members are not getting any of the inherent benefits of sports participation and others are being over-worked and unduly pressured to perform.

Team practices serve to keep the athletes in peak shape between competitions. They build speed, agility, endurance, muscular strength, and cardiovascular fitness. The repetitive drills aid in building the brain-to-body functions involved in fine motor coordination and concentration. Because all these aspects of sports play are vital to healthy competition, many teams are now imposing the safety rule: "No practice, no play." If your child's coach doesn't enforce this, you should make it a nonnegotiable family rule. Practice does make perfect; it also makes your young athlete less prone to injury.

To help athletes maintain a high level of skill performance during the off- and pre-season, many parents send their children to sport camps. Quality camps that are run by professional sports figures generally focus on proper technique and basic skill development to improve sports play and reduce the risk of injury. Ideally, these camps promote the true goals of athletics which include enjoyment of the sport with equal participation opportunities for all. If your young athlete has the chance to attend such a camp, it will most likely enhance his or her knowledge, skill level, and therefore enjoyment of the sport.

Evaluating the Coaches

At any level of play and in any sport, a parent's best ally in the fight against sports-related injuries is a coach who is educated about first aid as well as safe training, sound conditioning practices, and sports psychology. Although it has been found that the potential for injury may be greater for athletes who are instructed by coaches without this knowledge, unfortunately there is no nationally accepted system of certification for coaches in the U.S. In fact, of the 3.5 million coaches involved in youth athletics, probably fewer than 20 percent of them have received any formal training to become a coach.[1] This problem exists in both youth and high school sports programs because too often the demand for coaches exceeds the supply. As a result, athletic directors must fill coaching positions with inexperienced, unqualified (albeit well-meaning) individuals.

What this means is that to protect your child adequately from sports-related injuries, you must stand on the sidelines and monitor the coaching situation. To begin your evaluation, talk to the team coaches. Find out if the team has an athletic trainer. Trainers are becoming more commonplace within high school sports programs and even in some youth leagues. These professionals detect and treat the safety and health problems of over-training, fatigue, and injury, freeing coaches to concentrate fully on their jobs.

Next, ask the coaches about their philosophies and experiences. This doesn't need to be an interrogation; you can squeeze it into casual conversation with questions like, "How long have you been coaching?" and, "So, do you think we'll have a winning season?" If you find a coach who is inexperienced or who has a winning record to uphold, you should probably keep a closer watch on the methods of instruction. These individuals may ask young athletes to perform on a level that is inappropriate for their age and physical development, or they may bully them into long, relentless practice sessions. Young athletes who are expected to perform like older athletes or are pushed beyond their capabilities to the point of continual fatigue are more liable to injury and to sports burnout.

When you observe team practices, you'll have an opportunity to see if the philosophy of competition advocated by the coach in conversation is the same one he or she conveys to the players. If the coach persistently belittles, embarrasses, or scolds the athletes, and places a higher priority on winning than on proper technique and good sportsmanship, he or she is endangering your child's physical and mental health. Don't kid yourself by pretending that if your children want to play sports, they've got to be tough and learn to take it. There are many good coaches who teach, guide, encourage, and support without endangering the players' love of the sport or their physical well-being. On all levels of play the athletes' welfare should be the number one concern of all coaches.

It's usually true that younger athletes need more specific skill training and encouragement than high school athletes, who can be trained and pushed with more disciplined intensity. On any level, however, boot-camp-like routines can jeopardize young athletes' vulnerable growth zones and positive attitudes toward sports. The following questions will help you evaluate your child's coach:

1. Do the attitudes and actions of this coach provide a good role model?
2. Is this coach knowledgeable about the rules and proper techniques of this sport?
3. Is this coach able to help young athletes improve their skills?
4. Does this coach know what to do when an athlete is injured?
5. Is this the kind of coach whose reputation for winning would never take precedence over the well-being of the athletes?

6. Does this coach make an effort to reassure an athlete who has made a mistake?
7. Does this coach use positive motivation techniques such as praise, encouragement, and rewards more often than negative ones such as threats, ridicule, and punishments?

If you find more "no" than "yes" answers to these questions, it is very likely that your young athlete will not have a positive experience in sports and runs an increased risk of sustaining a sports-related injury.

If your child's team is led by this kind of coach, what can you do? Obviously, you want your children to play, you want them to finish the season, and you don't want them to be penalized by a vindictive coach if you complain. You may feel as though you're caught between allowing a bad situation to continue or yanking your child off the team. The following section will help you find an acceptable route out of this predicament.

Flexing Your Parent Power

When your athlete joins a team, introduce yourself to the coaches and express a positive attitude that says, "I'm looking forward to an enjoyable and injury-free season, and I know that together we can achieve this goal." Let them know right from the start that you support good coaching and safe athletics. This is also the time to express your concerns and ask questions about equipment quality and fit, skill instruction, and body conditioning. Once you've established that these things are important to you, it will be easier to pursue them if they are neglected later in the season.

Many coaches will take your interest in sports enjoyment and safety as a gentle reminder of what is really important in youth and high school sports. Coaches have reason to worry that their competency is calculated only by the number of games won. Let them know that most parents realize there is more to sports than just winning. When you feel the coaches are doing a good job, say so. Compliment their efforts and write letters to the league and local papers pinpointing what parents expect from and appreciate in athletics. This public approval will make it easier and more acceptable for all coaches to put fun and safety over winning.

Other coaches, however, who do not see health and enjoyment as priorities, put young athletes at risk for injury and burnout. When this happens you may feel uncomfortable complaining about situations that no one else seems to mind, or you may worry that if you raise a ruckus you'll appear overprotective. That's why your job of protecting the health of young athletes will be easier and more productive if you work with other parents to support good coaching and demand programs that emphasize safe athletics. If you find unsafe conditions or unacceptable training regimens and coaching techniques, it is most likely that others have noticed them too and together you *can* change them.

As a group, bring your concerns to the attention of the coach. Approach him or her with an attitude that says, "Like you, we all want our kids to play in a safe and healthy environment. So we'd like you to rethink the way this program is being handled." You may find that an honest, calm discussion between parents and coaches is all that's needed to change potentially dangerous situations into safe ones.

If, however, a coach refuses to recognize your concerns, or if the solution to the problem is out of his or her hands (such as a safe playing location), then bring your concerns to the person in charge of that local league. Whatever sport your children play, you can be sure that the league was originally organized with good intentions, and if parents present a unified front, their concerns will probably not be ignored. After all, the team exists to serve the positive development of the kids. If this is not happening, and those in charge will not take steps to ensure that it does, the entire program is in jeopardy. The ultimate option for concerned parents is to contact the national governing body of the sport program (see the listing of such organizations in Appendix B), and remove their children from the team. You can't claim to be interested in preventing injuries and then just ignore dangerous situations: make an effort to rectify the problem or find a safer league or sport.

You may find that it takes a significant amount of money to correct some potentially injurious conditions, such as worn equipment. A fund-raiser sponsored by a parent booster club may be the answer. Throughout the country, bake sales, car washes, candy and magazine drives have financed safe, appropriate facilities and equipment for thousands of young athletes.

A unified parent group may also be able to convince area coaches to become trained and certified through one of the programs listed in Appendix B. This will reduce the risk of injury to the athletes, but as an additional selling point, it may reduce the cost of insurance. The National Youth Sports Coaches Association, for example, provides a $500,000 liability insurance policy for each of the coaches it certifies.

As parents of young athletes, your role is to build injury prevention into the foundation of the sports program by providing support, good example, and sideline monitoring. For millions of kids each year, the sports experience is a good one, and the coaches, officials, parents, and athletes deserve credit for these successes. However, if dangerous conditions exist on any playing field in America, the blame must be shared by the parents for allowing it to continue.

2

■■■■■

The Daily Ingredients of Good Health—Diet and Rest

As a caring parent you certainly know that growing kids need well-balanced, nutritious, and varied daily diets as well as a good night's sleep. As the parent of a young athlete, you may have additional concerns: Does your child need different foods or more sleep than a non-athlete? How do you create and maintain a healthy regime? This chapter will explain what young athletes need to eat, how to plan a menu around these needs, and how their diets and sleep patterns should compare to those of non-athletes.

Diet

A typical day in the Lane household hardly leaves time for three meals on the run, never mind a family dinner hour that would give 12-year-old Danielle and 10-year-old John home-cooked samplings from the four basic food groups. As in many families, both parents work and the kids are involved in sports.

This means that the entire family is rarely together at home until after nine o'clock at night.

Danielle is a promising gymnast. She practices four days a week from 7 to 9 P.M. and often competes on weekends. John is a shortstop on his baseball team in the spring, a wide receiver on the football team in the fall, and a lightweight wrestler in the winter. He practices or competes five to six days a week, usually from 3:30 to 6:30 P.M. His parents get home at 6:30 each night—just in time to pick John up and drop Danielle off. In a brief exchange of how-do-you-do's, the question "Did you eat something?" usually comes up. "Yeah" is always the answer. Maybe a better question would be "WHAT did you eat?"

Danielle wants to lose weight because she thinks it will make her a better gymnast. She eats a quick breakfast because her mom insists that she put something in her stomach, but she skips lunch completely, and grabs a yogurt or an apple before she leaves for practice. John wants to gain weight so he'll be tougher in football and can move up one weight class in wrestling. Throughout the day he stuffs himself with cakes and candy. He has begun begging his parents to buy him a liquid supplement that the advertisement in his sports magazine says will "add pounds in just days."

Danielle and John are existing on substandard diets that jeopardize their health and athletic performance, yet they are not neglected kids and the Lanes are not uncaring parents. In fact, their diets typify those of many sports-involved families. Unfortunately, when these kinds of hit-or-miss diets become the standard, the kids become more prone to injury; to stay strong their growing bodies need more than yogurts and cakes, and even more than hot dogs, hamburgers, and pizza.

Danielle and John don't need super-nutritious meals because they are athletes, but we are often led to believe they do. Many advertisements claim the necessity of "super strength and energy diets"; stories about some pro athletes suggest success depends on eating five steaks and two raw eggs every day; myths persist that high-protein diets and special salt-laden drinks improve athletic performance. The truth is that athletes of all ages need the same well-balanced, varied diet that all people require. In fact, with the exception of additional calories and fluids, anyone who alters a daily diet to take in more of one food component than another risks upsetting the body's natural balance. Too much calcium, for example, may lead to an iron deficiency; an excess of phosphorus may limit the body's ability to absorb iron; and an overabundance of protein can cause dehydration, appetite loss, and diarrhea.

Diet is one area of injury prevention where you can have complete control and effect positive results in a short period of time with just a bit of knowledge and advanced planning. You don't need to create a super-powered diet plan; you simply need to know the kinds of foods that all kids require and make those available to your children. The following sections of this chapter will give you information about the dietary needs of your young athlete. It will also note problem diet situations, such as losing or gaining pounds to "make weight," the use of commercial supplements, and the development of eating disorders.

Four Food Groups

All children need a diet that includes daily portions from the four main food groups. Even though sports season is a busy time, it really is not difficult to calculate nutrients and analyze food composition and it plays an important role in deterring sports injuries. If you provide the minimal number of servings from each of the four food groups listed below, your young athlete will have a well-balanced diet that will provide the nutrients necessary for optimal health and maximum athletic performance.

To feed young athletes properly, you don't need to make special recipes, completely change your eating style, or spend extra money at health food stores. You just need to plan ahead. An example of a menu for an ordinary day might be:

CHART 2.1
AVERAGE DAILY MEAL

	Dairy	Meat	Fr/Veg	Grain
Breakfast:				
orange juice			1	
cereal (non-sugared is best)				1
with milk	1			
Lunch:				
peanut butter and jelly				
sandwich		1	1	1
glass of milk	1			
apple			1	
Snack:				
fruit juice			1	
oatmeal cookies				1
Dinner:				
cold chicken (cooked in large sup-				
ply on the weekend and refriger-				
ated for quick meals)		1		
a slice of wheat bread				1
carrot sticks			1	
Dessert:				
frozen yogurt	1			
Total:	3	2	5	4

To see how much adjusting you need to do in your planning, shopping, and cooking routines, make a list of all the foods your athlete will eat today. Check them against the requirements of the four food groups listed on following page. This will tell you something about the quality of present food intake and the steps you need to take to gear up for an optimal daily diet.

The Six Components of Food

Every day your athlete needs the proper mix of six food components: protein, carbohydrates, fat, vitamins, minerals,

CHART 2.2
FOUR FOOD GROUPS

Dairy	Meat	Fruits and Vegetables	Grains
2 servings	2 servings	4 servings	4 servings
milk	beef	all fruits	breads
cheese	pork	all vegetables	cereal
ice cream	lamb	fruit juices	spaghetti
cottage cheese	fish	tomatoes	noodles
pudding	poultry	salad greens	pancakes
creamed soups	eggs	cabbage	muffins
yogurt	peanut butter	potatoes	rice
	nuts		

and water. In a daily diet that includes foods from the four food groups listed above, these components occur naturally and in plentiful supply. That's why it's quite unnecessary for you to break down everything your children eat to verify that they're getting the required 40 percent protein, 45 percent carbohydrates, and 15 percent fat each day. The following information on the six components explains why some foods in the four food groups are better than others, and emphasizes why haphazard diets detract from your child's performance in and enjoyment of sports.

Protein

Protein is vital for body growth and injury repair. This is because it's an essential component of each and every cell in the body, making up 20 percent of the total cell mass. In addition, it's necessary for the development of muscle and internal bone structure. Protein exists in high quantities in fish, fowl, red meats, cow's milk and cheeses, to some degree in vegetables (especially beans and peas), and in trace amounts in fruits.

It was once believed that to build muscles and body strength athletes needed to increase their protein intake. Now we know that this is not true. Not only does excess protein *not* help athletes improve their performance, it can endanger their health. Those who increase their intake usually exclude other foods that are necessary to healthy body functioning. To compound that problem, when they surpass the body's daily requirements they risk developing painful and debilitating kidney stones.

There is no reason for athletes to increase their protein intake; a balanced diet supplies the human body with an ample supply of this vital food component. If a coach recommends a high-protein diet, he or she is perhaps well-meaning, but unaware of the latest medical research findings. This is another instance where you won't overstep your parental bounds by refusing to accept a high-protein diet.

Carbohydrates

Just before competitions, Olympic-level athletes often eat foods high in carbohydrates—the body's primary source of quick energy. Because your child needs such peak levels of energy and high caloric intake each day, foods with carbohydrates are important not only before sport competitions, but in the regular diet as well.

You should know, however, that carbohydrates come in two forms. *Simple* carbohydrates are found in sugar products such as table sugar, honey, candy, soda, and cake. These are quickly digested and absorbed through the body and give a quick but temporary energy boost. Following this initial lift, however, the sugar level in the blood drops below normal and causes body weakness, fatigue, and quickened heart rate. That's why sports workout after a dinner of cookies (even though they contain carbohydrates) is difficult and dangerous.

The second form, *complex* carbohydrates, also gives the body energy, but rather than a quick boost, it provides a long-term energy source that can prolong an athlete's ability to function at optimal levels. Complex carbohydrates are found in starches. Convenient sources include whole wheat breads, low-sugar cereals, pasta, and rice; vegetables, especially potatoes, sweet potatoes, lima beans, peas, corn, winter squash, carrots, and beets; fruit juices and fruits such as apples and oranges; and nuts such as peanuts and almonds.

The body will look to carbohydrates for its energy, but if there aren't enough in the diet, the body will take its energy from the protein in the muscles and other tissues. When this happens protein is less available to build muscle tissue and promote health. That, of course, opens the body to injury.

If your young athlete has low-sugar cereal for breakfast (or pancakes, waffles, or whole wheat toast), an apple with lunch, and a handful of peanuts before sports practice, he or she will have enough carbohydrates to increase the store of energy in the muscles, gain endurance, and spare protein for its job in muscle growth and repair.

Fats

Fats are an essential component of your young athlete's diet. They are found in every body cell, and they aid in the absorption of vitamins A, D, E, and K. They are a highly concentrated energy source, and they are a readily available source of calories.

As valuable a food element as fat is, however, most American diets overemphasize fast foods, processed foods, and junk foods which are too high in fat content. A McDonald's Big Mac, for example, contains 52 percent fat, a Burger King Whopper, 48 percent; both Dairy Queen Brazier Onion Rings and a Kentucky Fried Chicken Extra Crispy Dinner ring in at 51 percent.

An occasional fast-food meal will not destroy a good diet, especially if you know how to balance it with less fatty meals during the day. When choosing from the four food groups listed earlier, try to avoid a high concentration of these fatty substances:

1. red meats (steak, hamburger, hot dogs, luncheon meats, and so forth)
2. pork products (bacon and sausage)
3. whole milk, ice cream, cream sauces
4. cheese
5. butter or margarine
6. mayonnaise or salad dressing
7. cooking oils
8. salad dressings
9. french fries and potato chips

When your athlete does eat these foods, you can lower the fat content by following these guidelines:

1. Buy lean cuts of meat and trim all excess fat.
2. Keep meats to moderate servings and substitute fish and poultry.
3. Remove the skin from fish and poultry; it is nearly 100 percent fat.
4. Don't fry foods: bake, broil, boil, poach, steam, barbecue.
5. Switch to skim milk or low-fat milk.
6. Avoid foods packed in oil.

Vitamins and Minerals

Vitamins and minerals are chemical substances necessary for normal body growth and functioning. They are, however, not manufactured by the body, but found only in the foods we eat. Although they don't contain energy and are not used for fuel, they help regulate the rate at which chemical reactions, such as calcium absorption, occur. Minerals are found in the earth. We get our supply of them by eating plants which absorb them from the soil, or the animals which assimilate them from plants or other animals. Minerals are needed to control the heartbeat, contract the muscles, and conduct nerve impulses.

The body depends on a full supply of vitamins and minerals to work at peak levels. Although the body's daily requirements for these two components vary depending on a person's state of health, body size, age, state of growth, and sex, a daily diet including foods from the four food groups will give your athlete all he or she needs.

Still, many parents worry that on-the-run sport dinners aren't enough to keep young athletes fully supplied with this important nutrient duo. So with good intentions, they attempt to fill the vitamin/mineral gap with supplements. This may appear to be a harmless precaution to parents who believe that the body will take what it needs from pills and excrete the excess amounts. Although this is true of some vitamins and minerals, there are others that are not water soluble and therefore can not be broken down and processed through the kidney and into the urine. These vitamins (A, D, E, K) and minerals (such as calcium, magnesium, and potassium) are toxic in high doses and can do substantial harm to a young athlete's growing body. If you give your child a daily multiple vitamin/mineral complex that supplies only the recommended daily amounts, you will not cause him or her any harm, but your money would be better spent on nutritious foods. Under no circumstances, however, should a healthy athlete under the age of 18 take high doses of particular vitamins or minerals in an effort to improve physical performance.

Water

Water is absolutely essential for optimal athletic performance. Unlike the need for protein, carbohydrates, fats, vitamins, and minerals, which remains constant even in the off-season, the athlete's requirements for water exceed those of the non-athlete. Strenuous and intense activity rapidly depletes the supply of fluids needed to continually move nutrients and oxygen throughout the body. A full supply of water is especially necessary during exercise because the muscles generate a massive amount of heat which must be transported by body fluids to the skin's surface. There it is dissipated as sweat.

Before adolescence, children do not perspire efficiently. However, they are less likely than older athletes to recognize the symptoms of dehydration, less likely to complain, and less likely to take in the fluids they need during practice or competitions. For these reasons, if your athlete is in a youth league, you may want to be particularly vigilant in monitoring water intake. Regardless of your child's age or sport, make sure he or she knows the importance of drinking lots of water and can recognize the warning signs of dehydration.

These warning signs include:

- rise in pulse rate
- fatigue
- muscle cramps
- decrease in ability to perform up to par
- headaches or nausea (signs of heat exhaustion)
- extremely high body temperature without sweating, hot flushed skin, confusion, or even unconsciousness (signs of heat stroke)

The easiest way to deal with dehydration is to prevent it. Make sure your athlete knows he or she must drink 8 to 10 ounces of cool water before practice or competition and again every 25 minutes during play in hot weather. (Cool water is best because it is absorbed faster by the body and is less likely than warm water to cause cramps.)

A number of drinks, powders, and tablets are sometimes offered by coaches and teammates to replace the salt and electrolytes that are lost through sweat. At best, these supplements are useless because the balanced diet that meets an athlete's energy needs also provides all the salts, minerals, and electrolytes utilized during strenuous workouts. At worst, they are dangerous because they make it more difficult for the body to maintain a healthy balance of these elements. They can also fill the stomach, causing the athlete to feel bloated and can mask the athlete's thirst and need for water. Make sure that your child knows that "sports drinks" or salt tablets do *not* replace the body's need for water.

After physical activity, water is needed to give back to the body what it lost through sweat. Encourage your child to make a habit of drinking it throughout each day. Also, monitor water intake by keeping track of his or her weight. If an athlete drops weight during the sports season, it is a sign that more calories should be included in the daily diet (preferably through complex carbohydrates), but it's also a warning sign that the water lost during physical activity is not being replenished. A drop of even two or three percent of total body weight from water loss (from 110 pounds to less than 108, for example) will increase body temperature and pulse rate, promote fatigue, and decrease performance ability.

Water is a mode of injury prevention that is simple, inexpensive, and readily available. Tape a sign over your kitchen sink that says, "Have a glass of water!"

Eating Before Athletic Events

Athletic performance can't be enhanced with a nutritious pre-game meal. The foods that are needed to perform at optimal levels must be eaten during the entire week before the big event. For best results, serve a light pre-game meal at least three hours before activity. This is because during normal digestion the heart pumps large amounts of blood to the gastrointestinal tract. When active muscles call for more blood, the supply to the digestive system is slowed, leaving undigested foods that can cause cramps.

Because complex carbohydrates are a good source of quick and yet long-lasting energy, an early meal of cooked pasta and vegetables with a fruit and gelatin dessert is ideal. Be sure also to include several glasses of water.

Athletes who get hungry between matches, meets, or games should eat light snacks of oranges, raisins, and bananas. But they should avoid sugary snacks of simple carbohydrates like candy bars and cookies because, although they give a quick energy boost, the sugar level may drop down before it's time to compete. When this happens, not only does diet detract from performance, it works against the athlete by causing feelings of fatigue and sluggishness.

If, because of your family schedule, it's impossible to get nutritious foods into your young athlete three hours before activity, you might try substituting a liquid-drink meal. Although these should not routinely take the place of a nutritious diet, they are a good option for the child who might otherwise choose a piece of cake or nothing at all. Products such as Sustacal® and Ensure® are nutritious liquid foods manufactured for people who must live on a liquid diet. Ask your doctor or pharmacist to recommend one.

Making Weight

The foods we eat work most efficiently to give the body strength and energy when weight is kept within the "normal" range. Athletes such as gymnasts, dancers, figure skaters, distance runners, cross-country skiers, and those in endurance sports know that excess body fat limits their performance abilities. Other activities, such as wrestling, boxing, and junior league football, require athletes to "weigh-in" and to compete within their own weight category. Some athletes (especially young, thin ones) believe that *extra* pounds will enhance their performance in contact sports like football and soccer. Unfortunately, sometimes kids lose sight of what's "normal" for their age and height, and so they go through extreme weight alteration programs in an attempt to attain the perfect weight for their sport.

Although most coaches today know the dangers of these extreme methods, young athletes are still apt to follow the advice and example of peers who push dehydration diets to lose weight rapidly and gimmicky high-calorie systems to put on quick pounds. To prevent serious injury and illness, you should step in immediately to stop any diet that drastically limits or increases the intake of the foods discussed in this chapter.

Because altering body weight and composition to compete in sports is quite common, very dangerous, and sometimes the precursor to anabolic steroid use and eating disorders (such as anorexia and bulimia), the subject is discussed at length in Chapter Five, "The Dangerous Side of Sports Play."

Sleep

Young athletes often live hectic and hurried lives. After school they have homework to do, chores to finish, and meals to eat; they attend sports practice and competitions and seem to need an obligatory dose of TV watching and video game playing. When there's too much to do in one day, or when a sporting event runs late, it's an athlete's sleep needs that often get pushed aside.

Nine-year-old Matt amazed his family with his endless supply of energy. He was able to rise each morning at 7:00 to finish homework, eat, wash, dress, and get out of the house to catch the school bus at 7:45. After a full day of school, he would run in the back door of his house, jump into his play clothes, and dash back out to soccer practice. At 6:00 each night, he'd rush back into the house to grab a quick bite to eat, shower, change his clothes, and do some homework. At 9:00, Matt would say goodnight to his parents and spend the next hour reading or watching TV in his room. When wrestling season began, his parents worried that Matt was doing too much, so they suggested that he go to sleep earlier. But because his school grades were good and he seemed perfectly healthy, they gave in, with misgivings, to Matt's pleading and let him run his daily race to a 10:00 P.M. bedtime finish each night.

Like many children between the ages of six and twelve, Matt falls asleep easily, sleeps soundly, and is on the go without signs of sleepiness throughout the day. Children in this age group can generally go to bed between eight and ten o'clock at night, get up between six and eight in the morning and be completely rested.

Surprisingly, teenagers generally need more sleep than younger children, and they experience more frequent episodes of daytime fatigue. Although some teens are tired because they don't get the recommended eight to ten hours of sleep each night, studies have found that even when allowed to sleep as long as they like, adolescents tend to be sleepy during the day.

Daytime lethargy may occur as the body instinctively seeks the growth hormones that are secreted during sleep; since the teen years are a time of rapid physical development, their bodies may crave sleep to fulfill a biological need. This makes it difficult to determine if teen athletes are tired because they are not getting enough sleep or simply because they are teenagers.

Although sleep requirements vary among individuals and also depend on age, and physical and emotional health, most teens need *at least* eight hours of sleep each night. Use this amount as a general gauge. If your adolescent athlete isn't getting eight hours of sleep each night, sleep deprivation is to blame for the feelings of fatigue. If after a full night's sleep he or she is still tired, active growth hormones may be the culprit.

Whether your children want to or not, sleep is something they can not decide to skip. In fact, like it or not, the average person spends one-third of a lifetime sleeping. This need affects athletes and non-athletes alike. According to *The American Medical Association Straight-talk, No-nonsense Guide to*

Better Sleep, very active people don't, on the average, need any more or less sleep than non-active people: professional athletes get the same amount of sleep as their fans.

The human body is able to adjust to occasional changes in sleep patterns. If, for example, your children stay up past midnight because they have pre-game jitters, or late-night games, or extraordinarily long homework assignments, the few hours of lost sleep should affect neither their performance the next day nor their overall health. If, however, young athletes continually fall short of the needed eight to ten hours of sleep, their bodies will begin to react to the deficit and they will become more prone to injury. Lack of sleep over an extended period of time will make children sluggish and tired, and it will also make it difficult for them to concentrate and stay alert. All of these conditions are obviously dangerous to an athlete because safe sports-play requires ready energy, sharp reflexes, and quick thinking.

You can help your young athlete remain healthy through the sports season by establishing a nightly bedtime. You might say, for example, "If you are going to be involved in this sport, then you have to agree that you will be in bed with the lights out by 10:00 every night." This will eliminate the bad habits of watching late-night TV, putting off homework until after 10:00, and talking on the telephone until all hours. If a sound sleep routine is followed throughout the season, your young athlete will have no trouble dealing with the loss of sleep that can occasionally occur because of sports involvement.

Good diets and appropriate sleep patterns are important aspects of any injury prevention program. As parents, you are in a good position to make sure that before your young athletes go out to compete, they have the strong and healthy bodies they need. The next chapter will explain how you can complement these efforts by overseeing a conditioning program that improves flexibility, agility, speed, cardiovascular and muscular endurance, and strength.

3

■ ■ ■ ■ ■

Body Conditioning

All athletes are not created equal. Some are better basketball players because of their height; others excel as
dancers because they're agile and lean; still others are star
sprinters because they're fast. There are several reasons why
some kids are "natural" athletes.

Some people are actually "made" in ways that enhance
sports participation. Their muscles hold more oxygen, and so
they don't tire as quickly as others. Certain people have more
of a particular type of muscle fiber that enables them to run
faster than others. Their bodies can more quickly and efficiently turn sugar into energy: these are the star sprinters.
You can observe these natural athletes on the first day of
sports practice. Look around and you'll notice that without
any training, conditioning, or coaching, there's always a kid
who jumps higher than anyone else or runs laps without ever
getting tired. These athletes come to the game with a physical
advantage.

The majority of children, however, need to train their bodies
to perform athletic feats; this body training, called conditioning, should be age-appropriate and, ideally, is an integral part
of all athletic programs. It keeps athletes in shape for their
sports and it improves their ability to play. This, in turn,

enhances their enjoyment of the sport and greatly reduces the likelihood of incurring a sports-related injury.

Age Considerations

A conditioning program for the youth-league player (ages 5 to 12 or 13) differs in many ways from one for the adolescent athlete. The American College of Sports Medicine recommends that children engage in 20 to 30 minutes of exercise activity each day to develop and maintain the ability to promote optimal health and to meet the physical demands of a growing individual. Children who participate in daily gym classes and outdoor play can generally meet these guidelines with ease. However, studies have repeatedly shown that younger athletes do not benefit from rigorous, regimented, or intense physical routines. In fact, overuse injuries such as stress fractures and sprains are commonly found in youngsters who work out more than three to five times each week and don't get a chance to rest between training periods to allow for physiological as well as psychological adjustment. Young athletes develop best under the "not too much and not to soon" rule. Because their musculoskeletal system is still growing, the growth plates are open and they're still building body strength. Therefore, these kids need conditioning practice sessions that stress warm-ups, proper technique, cool-down periods, and above all, fun. This kind of conditioning program will build the training habits that prepare young athletes for the more intense workouts that will be most beneficial to them in high school sports.

In addition to the warm-up/cool-down program of younger athletes, high school competitors are physically ready to benefit from a wider range of conditioning exercises. Male athletes, for example, whose testosterone hormone production enables them to build muscle mass, more readily profit from strength training. For both sexes, aerobic capabilities continue to increase the more children engage in cardiovascular exercise. Adolescents and teens undergoing growth spurts often lose muscle flexibility and need stretching exercises to keep muscles loose. (See Chapter Fifteen for a full discussion of the physical changes that occur during growth spurts.) Because high school sports programs tend to be highly competitive and strenuous, body conditioning figures prominently in injury prevention, while younger athletes can prepare for teen sports by establishing good training habits now.

Adaption

The body of a couch potato performs at relatively low levels. When this slow-motion person decides to jump into action, the body can *adapt* itself to the call for additional energy and strength—as long as it is given a period of transitional conditioning.

The undisciplined body's first response to even mild sudden activity may come in the form of sore muscles, shortness of breath, cramps, blisters, and stiffness. But as it is progressively trained to work harder, physiology changes in ways that allow for increasing degrees of intense activity without discomfort. The circulatory system learns to widen the blood vessels to the working muscles where more blood is demanded and to narrow those leading to other organs not in immediate need. This "shunting" or directing of blood is a protective mechanism controlled by the brain. When a person goes into shock, for example, the skin and muscles seem very cool because the blood has been shunted away from the musculoskeletal system and the peripheral regions of the body to the kidneys and brain where it is most essential. During exercise, the blood is directed to the working muscles. With transitional conditioning, the nervous system learns to push more muscle fibers into action. The muscles respond to the call to action by converting carbohydrates into energy. The heart learns to pump harder without strain to give the muscles the extra oxygen they need. Bones, tendons, ligaments, and connective tissues strengthen and skin becomes tougher and builds calluses where needed.

Overload

The process of adaption works on a principle called *overload*. To understand this principle consider, for example, a track athlete, Janet, who wants to run cross country. Eventually she will run five miles with ease without suffering fatigue or muscle cramps, but on the first day of practice, Janet may be exhausted after running only one mile. The next day she will run the same distance (now with sore muscles and blistered feet), but she will probably feel less fatigue and pain. Each day this one-mile run will become easier as her body adapts to the call for extra strength and energy. Once this happens, Janet must overload her newly conditioned body and push it to adapt even further to run two miles. When those miles are run with relative ease, she will be ready to overload again and strive to a further distance. Overload conditioning and body adaption will improve physical performance when the body is progressively forced beyond the first signs of tiredness. Athletes must be careful, however, not to push beyond their top level of tolerance. This violates the principle of progression.

Progression

What would happen if long-distance hopeful, Janet, decided to run a brisk five miles on the first day of training without prior conditioning? Her body could not adapt to this sudden overload. It would respond with intense pain and fatigue. It's not that Janet can't run five miles, but simply that her body can't adapt so quickly.

Conditioning is a progressive process. Proper training slowly builds the body by overloading in small doses. At a slow pace an athlete can steadily increase the frequency, intensity, and length of training time. At first, there will be rapid changes in the body's ability to adjust to increased demands. With persistent conditioning, the mile run, for example, can be pushed to a two-mile run in just a few days. The jump from an easy seven-mile to an easy ten-mile run, however, will probably take more effort and longer training. It can be accomplished when athletes condition themselves according to the principles of adaption, overload, and progression.

Specificity

The kind of physical stress placed on athletes' bodies varies from one sport to another. Cross-country runners, for example, need endurance, while sprinters need speed; weightlifters need strength, and gymnasts need agility. Each can enhance performance by putting pre-season and in-season emphasis on the exercises that support the needs of the individual sport. Chart 3.1 on page 47 will give you some insight into specific conditioning requirements, while a list of training regimes most appropriate to each activity is included in Part II of this book.

Cross-training of all muscle groups during the off-season is recommended for young athletes. This will foster healthy growth and improve their general muscular development and balance.

Reverse Adaptability

Just as the body adapts to increased strength and energy, it also changes back to the pre-activity state when exercise stops. That's why the star basketball player, who could run up and down the court at the end of last season for two hours without feeling the least bit fatigued, will suffer from exhaustion and cramps after only thirty minutes of play on the first day of this season's practice.

As you can see, conditioning is a slow steady process that can't be rushed. But because there's little time between the first practice and the first game, young athletes commonly push their bodies to perform without allowing time for paced overload and progression. To avoid injuries that happen when they're out of shape, elementary school athletes should begin a relaxed conditioning regime several weeks before the first official practice. A program of warm-up exercises (page 44), flexibility stretches (page 65), light calisthenics or jogging, and a cool-down period (page 45) several days a week for only 15 to 20 minutes will substantially reduce their risk of an early season sports-related injury.

High school athletes often engage in more competitively intense sports activities. Their practices are sometimes organized around a "play-till-you-drop" philosophy, and there is little time for gradual conditioning. For this reason, year-round training programs are very important. The need for such a regime also applies to athletes who return to activity after a vacation break or go from one sport to another. They may find themselves fatigued and out of breath at the first practice if they haven't exercised the muscle groups used in that sport.

Most athletic trainers advise young competitors to develop a pre-, in-, post- and off-season conditioning program that varies in intensity, frequency, and specificity. Pre-season training should begin at least six weeks before the start of competition. It should work the body parts stressed by the particular sport (see Part II) and it should be practiced in intense hour-long workouts 3 to a maximum of 5 days a week. Once the sport season begins and athletes are involved in practice sessions that enhance their physical readiness to play, the training program should be reduced in intensity to 15 minutes 3 times a week; this will enable the athlete to maintain the level of conditioning that was attained during the pre-season sessions. Post-season is a time for 3 to 4 weeks of "active" rest. During this time youngsters should enjoy recreational activities such as bicycling, swimming, and jogging. Off-season, athletes should practice an exercise regime that gives them general, all-over body conditioning. This cross-training helps young athletes build muscle balance, maintain a base-level of fitness, and it also helps them establish life-long attitudes and health habits that make exercise an integral part of daily life.

Warm-Up/Cool-Down

At the start of a conditioning session and when athletes first walk onto the playing area, their muscles are cold. The fibers do not have the blood and oxygen supply they need to spring into action, and if they are forced to work in this state they are prone to fatigue and injury. Therefore, the goal of warm-up exercising is to increase the blood flow, and therefore the oxygen supply, to the muscles; this will warm them so they can safely move from a dormant to an active state. As an athlete begins such exercises, the body takes blood from resting pools throughout the system and directs it to the muscles. They, in turn, then have enough oxygen to withstand the high energy consumption brought on by exercise.

A typical warm-up session might begin with slow jogging, rope-jumping, or cycling to get the blood pumping. This is often followed by a series of light calisthenics such as jumping jacks, trunk twists, sit-ups, and/or push-ups. When the muscles warm up and become further oxygenated they are ready for stretching exercises which will improve flexibility.

Unfortunately, warmed muscles cool off quickly. They can return to their pre-activity state of inflexibility during even short rest periods and half-time breaks. The majority of muscle injuries occur when athletes return from the sidelines to active play without taking time to recondition the muscles. Make sure that your young athletes develop the warm-up habit during the first 10 to 15 minutes of training, before any sports play, and after every rest period.

In the same way, all athletes should finish conditioning sessions, practices, and games with a cool-down period. Active muscles need high levels of oxygen to stay strong and functioning. If the body abruptly stops moving, the extra supply of oxygen that the muscles required only seconds earlier is suddenly cut off, and the muscles are left with what's called an oxygen debt. The goal of a cool-down period is to supply the fatigued muscles with blood until they have covered that debt. Muscles also need a cool-down period to help them pump out fluids that build up during activity. Without the time to cool off slowly, muscles may cramp or spasm.

A few minutes of such exercise can also prevent long-range muscle fatigue, a phenomenon that can make an otherwise healthy athlete prone to injury. After a game, your child can simply repeat the warm-up routine, or jog once around the playing area. Even a walk back to the locker room can work. Gentle stretches are important and should include the groin (page 10), the Achilles tendon (page 68), and the hamstring muscles (page 66). Cool-down exercises should be habitual after every period of intense exertion. Make sure your young athlete knows that the body should not be asked to switch from a high-energy state to a complete standstill without a transitional cool-down period.

Six Components of Body Conditioning

Total fitness involves several types of body conditioning. This chapter will discuss the six that are commonly needed to prevent injuries and attain top youth athletic performance: flexibility, agility, speed, cardiovascular endurance, muscular endurance, and muscular strength.

Fitness in all six areas is an ideal goal for any athlete, but sometimes emphasis should be placed on strengthening the body parts and functions stressed by a particular sport. Part II of this book details conditioning exercises most appropriate for optimal performance in a variety of popular sports. The chart below will also give you an idea of which fitness components should be emphasized.

A few sample exercises for each type of conditioning regime are given at the end of this chapter. These exercises are limited in number and are included in this book only as an introduction to body conditioning. You can ask your child's coach to recommend others.

Flexibility

Flexibility can be most easily defined as the full range of possible movement in a joint (as in the hip joint) or series of joints (like the vertebral column).[1] Varying degrees of flexibility are required in all sports for fluid motion and for the prevention of soft-tissue injuries.

Age Considerations

Young children are naturally supple. Their bodies seem to bend and stretch like rubber bands, so flexibility training for youth-league athletes is not usually necessary. Stretching, however, should be routinely included in their warm-up sessions. If young athletes develop that habit before any physical exertion, they will not be sidelined by a muscle injury. This conditioning will, as they get older, better prepare them to handle the growth spurts that tighten muscles.

Girls between the ages of eleven and thirteen and boys between the ages of thirteen and sixteen go through growth spurts. These periods of rapid body changes alter the posture and tighten the muscles. During this time young athletes are especially prone to injuries caused by overexertion of the muscle joint or connective tissue. Exactly how this affects their athletic ability is explained in Chapter Fifteen.

Benefits

Overexertion injuries commonly occur when athletes jump into action with cold muscles. These injuries range from mild muscle strain to complete muscle rupture or tear and can bench a player for a few minutes or for the entire season. They can also keep an athlete from achieving top-level performance because once hurt, a player may be prone to injure

CHART 3.1
ATHLETIC FITNESS SCORING CHART

Sport	Fitness Components*						
	Muscle Strength	Muscle Power	Speed	Agility	Flexibility	Muscle Endurance	Cardio-respiratory Endurance
Baseball	2	3	3	2	2	1	1
Basketball	2	3	2	3	2	2	3
Football—linemen	4	3	2	2	2	2	1
backs and receivers	2	3	3	3	3	2	2
Soccer	2	2	2	3	3	3	3
Tennis	1	2	2	3	2	2	2
Alpine skiing	2	2	2	2	1	4	4
Cross-country skiing	1	1	1	1	1	4	4
Gymnastics	4	4	3	4	4	3	2
Cycling—sprints	3	3	4	2	1	2	2
distance	2	1	1	1	1	4	4
Swimming—sprints	3	3	3	2	3	1	1
distance	2	1	1	1	3	4	4
Track and field—							
sprints	3	3	4	2	3	1	2
distance running	1	1	1	1	1	4	4
throwing events	4	4	3	3	3	3	1
jumping events	2	4	3	2	3	2	2
Your Score							

*1—above average; 2—good; 3—very good; 4—excellent.

the damaged area again. In the majority of cases this class of injury can be prevented if athletes correctly and habitually stretch their muscles for at least five minutes in warm-ups before competition, during cool-down after competition, and as part of all conditioning and practice sessions.

In addition to injury prevention, flexibility exercises have other benefits. They can: 1) increase the range of motion, 2) reduce soreness and stiffness after exercise, 3) maximize speed through increased stride length, 4) hasten rehabilitation of injuries, and 5) enhance the athlete's ability to master the movement skills of the sport. These benefits give athletes the advantage in all sports, but are especially important in those that require more flexible movement than others. On Chart 3.1 on page 47, for example, you'll notice that, above all others, the gymnast needs a full range of flexibility, while the distance runner needs the least.

Training

As you work with your young athlete to develop a pre- and in-season conditioning program, remember that stretching exercises are quite specific to certain joints and body tissues. The swimmer, for example, needs one stretching exercise for the shoulders, another for the hips, and still another for the hamstring muscles. Part II will specify which body parts need flexibility training in each sport. The off-season training program should keep all joints supple for overall body flexibility.

Whatever sport your young athletes play, help them learn *how* to stretch so that flexibility conditioning helps rather than hurts them.

CORRECT STRETCHING TECHNIQUE
1. Ease into stretch position.
   Slowly push the muscle to stretch until you feel slight pain.
2. Hold that position for at least five seconds.
   During this time the particular joint is locked into a position that lengthens the muscles and connective tissues. This kind of exercise is called a static stretch.
3. Relax.
   Return to your pre-stretch position and let the muscle rest a few seconds before stretching it again.
4. DO NOT use bouncing or jerking motions.

Bouncing in and out of a stretch position is a form of exercise called ballistic stretching. This is not recommended as part of flexibility training because as muscles quickly contract over and over again, they may actually shorten rather than stretch. This can cause muscle tears and will defeat the purpose and preventative quality of the stretching exercise.

Sample flexibility conditioning exercises are presented on page 67.

Agility

Agility refers to one's ability to shift direction of movement rapidly without losing balance or sense of position. This skill is especially necessary in sports like soccer, football, and basketball: the athlete must veer from side to side when running to outmaneuver opponents. It's also important to the tennis player, who makes quick movements in short steps; agility enables the gymnast to maintain control and perform with smooth, balanced motion.

Agility is not a single skill, but rather a combination of speed, strength, quick reaction, balance, and coordination. It is primarily an inherited trait, but it can be improved through repetitive practice of the specific desired movement. Basketball players, for example, who want to improve their vertical leaps should make ten successive jumps from a standing position without stopping. On the last attempt, they should tap chalk-coated fingers against the wall at the highest point. During the next agility-conditioning session the player will try to beat that mark. The conditioning goal of this agility drill is to raise the jump height average over a period of time.

Each sport demands different kinds of agile maneuvering. Some are listed under each sport discussed in Part II, and you can also ask the coach to recommend others. Because agility drills enhance a variety of physical attributes, constant repetition of them will improve the youth athlete's overall performance.

Sample agility conditioning exercises are presented on page 71.

Speed

Athletes can be taught how to bat, throw, dribble, kick, dive, spike, and vault. But the ability to move quickly is genetically determined by factors such as type and number of muscle fibers. (See pages 52 and 57 for a complete discussion of fast- and slow-twitch muscle fibers.) Through speed-conditioning, however, athletes can improve their reaction time (the time needed to decide to make a move) and the efficiency of their fast movements.

Anaerobic Energy

To understand why conditioning for speed is very different than conditioning for any other kind of movement, you need to know something about the body's biomechanics. To begin, let's take a look at the kind of energy used for quick action.

Any sport that requires less than two minutes of speed

activity before allowing for a period of rest works on what is called anaerobic energy—meaning energy without oxygen. This short-burst kind of energy is stored in all the body's muscles and quickly meets immediate energy needs without waiting for delivery of extra oxygen. This is a vital function when an athlete sprints the 100-yard dash, swims the 200-meter breaststroke, plays a point in tennis, racketball, or volleyball, or runs into the end zone.

When the body first demands instant energy, a chemical within the muscle called ATP (adenosine triphosphate) converts to ADP (adenosine diphosphate) which releases immediate muscle energy for ten to fifteen seconds. A high jump or a run to first base depletes the muscle's supply of ATP. As that store is consumed, the glycogen-lactic acid system kicks in to provide energy. Glycogen is a carbohydrate that is stored in muscles and fuels about two minutes of muscle activity without relying on extra oxygen. If the tennis point should extend for more than that amount of time, the players will deplete their anaerobic energy supply and begin to feel fatigued. This is because the instant energy source is empty and also because during the conversion of glycogen to energy, lactic acid is produced as a waste product. This material is irritating to the muscles and, if it is not carried away fast enough, will cause fatigue and pain or discomfort.

All of this may sound a bit technical and far removed from the topic of speed, but in fact, it explains why conditioning can improve a person's ability to move quickly, even though genetic make-up primarily determines speed. Through anaerobic conditioning muscles can be trained to tolerate lactic acid and thereby avoid fatigue and cramping. Conditioning can also increase the enzymatic production of glycogen, which improves the muscles' ability to metabolize the painful, fatiguing lactic acid and to utilize energy better. In addition, anaerobic speed training develops fast-reacting muscle fibers.

Fast-Twitch Muscle Fibers

Every muscle in the body contains two kinds of muscle fibers. Slow-twitch fibers are slow-reacting and are called into action in a sporting event requiring muscular endurance (page 56). Fast-twitch fibers are used in physical movements that call for quick reaction and speed. They generate a large amount of force in a short period of time and then quickly fatigue. Consistently used by sprinters, jumpers, discus throwers, shot putters, and weightlifters who demand quick bursts of energy, they are also used for initial action during the anaerobic movements in sports such as tennis, volleyball, football, basketball, and baseball.

The number and quality of fast-twitch muscle fibers varies from one athlete to another due to genetic predetermination. It is not surprising that studies have found that world-class sprinters and power athletes generally have a higher ratio of fast-twitch to slow-twitch fibers.

Training

Your young athletes can't change the number of muscle fibers they were born with, but they can improve their speed performance. Several kinds of body conditioning exercises contribute to speed. Flexibility increases fluidity and efficiency of body movements; agility improves the ability to make quick directional changes, and muscular strength increases initial acceleration speed. In addition, speed conditioning exercises like those listed at the end of this chapter can enhance anaerobic functioning while developing the fast-twitch fibers. Both of these body mechanisms dictate an athlete's potential for speed.

Sample speed conditioning exercises are presented on page 71.

Cardiovascular Endurance

Cardiovascular endurance is the ability of the circulatory, respiratory, and muscular systems to supply the body with energy for long periods of physical activity. This kind of endurance determines how far the distance runner, swimmer, or skier can go without becoming exhausted.

Aerobic Energy

Endurance athletes can't rely on the anaerobic energy system to keep them going because, as explained above, this system, which uses stored carbohydrates for energy, supplies only a one- to two-minute energy burst. Athletes involved in sports that demand muscle action for longer than that depend on oxygen for sustained energy; this is called the aerobic system of energy production. How well the aerobic system fuels an athlete depends on how efficiently the body can take in oxygen from the air, transport it to the lungs, and then deliver it through the bloodstream to the working muscles.

The amount of aerobic energy athletes receive to power their actions varies from one individual to another. Medical researchers have found that a person's upper limit of aerobic capacity is an inherited trait. But they have also discovered that most people need aerobic conditioning to reach that ceiling of energy production.

Maximal oxygenation (VO_2 max) is a term used to label a person's highest attainable oxygen uptake rate during exhaustive exercise.[2] The greater a person's concentration of oxygen (VO_2 max), the better his or her ultimate capacity for prolonged exercise. In children, VO_2 max increases for both sexes until the age of eight. Girls then steadily lose VO_2 max after this time, but it continues to increase in boys until the age of 16. (This is believed to be due to the relatively large amount of body fat in females compared to males.) That fact suggests that young girls may have greater need for aerobic conditioning than boys whose cardiovascular endurance continues to develop on its own.

An athlete's VO_2 max can be evaluated by measuring how much air is inhaled and how much air is exhaled during exhaustive exercise. In a variety of ways a doctor, coach, or athletic trainer can calculate a child's innate ability to use oxygen in energy production precisely. The most popular method of testing requires the athlete to run a treadmill or ride a stationary bicycle while he or she breathes through a mouth piece. Intake is then measured as oxygen enters this tube and the expired air is diverted to a gas meter which measures total volume and carbon dioxide and oxygen content. Comparative testing of VO_2 max can evaluate the progress of aerobic training and determine when an athlete has reached the limit of his or her cardiovascular endurance.

All athletes require above-average cardiovascular endurance, but especially those involved in sports that demand sustained action, such as soccer and basketball, or prolonged muscle movement, as in cross-country track, distance swimming, and cycling. Although the ability to produce energy to support the demands of these sports is affected by factors such as age, sex, health status, and heredity, endurance-event athletes past the age of puberty need training to reach their full potential.

Training

Cardiovascular endurance training strives first to improve the ability of the heart, blood vessels, blood, and lungs to supply oxygen to the muscles and then to increase the muscles' ability to turn that oxygen into energy. Through training, a number of bodily changes occurs that help the muscles do this efficiently:

1. an increase in the number of blood vessels

As muscles grow larger and stronger, extra blood vessels

develop to increase the amount of oxygenated blood they can deliver to these muscles.

2. improved performance of red blood cells
   Red blood cells increase the efficiency with which they carry the oxygen to the muscles. This increases the body's ability to fuel the muscles with energy.
3. enhanced lung capacity
   As the body learns to take in more oxygen with each breath, the lungs respond by enlarging their surface area. This allows more oxygen to be picked up by the red blood cells.
4. stronger chest muscles
   Aerobic training continually strengthens the chest muscles as they move the diaphragm in and out for respiration. The lungs therefore receive more air with each breath.

These four bodily changes help an athlete maximize oxygen intake per breath and distribute it more effectively with each heart beat. By enhancing the respiratory, circulatory, and muscular systems in this way, endurance training also contributes to the goal of injury prevention during sports play. If your athlete's body is not trained to withstand the demands of an endurance activity, he or she will quickly suffer from fatigue, shortness of breath, and muscle cramps. This in turn increases the likelihood of sustaining injury.

Aerobic training for cardiovascular stamina is an important part of a conditioning program for all athletes. Those competing in endurance events will obviously benefit from increased aerobic capacity. But even athletes who compete in sports that rely on the quick burst of energy supplied by anaerobic sources will find that aerobic training will help them recover quickly between events and will decrease bouts of fatigue that detract from practice time.

Like all kinds of conditioning, cardiovascular endurance exercises work best when used according to the principles of overload and progression. Start slowly. Then, as the body adapts to the call for more oxygen and the more efficient transport of the oxygen to the muscles, gradually and steadily add on to the exercise regime. For example, long-distance running effectively builds cardiovascular endurance. However, athletes should not expect to run a half-mile on the first day, a full mile on the second, and a mile-and-a-half on the third. A better and healthier progression is to begin with the goal of a comfortably paced quarter-mile for one week; increase that to a mile the following week, and continue adding on distance that is no greater than 20 percent of the week's total distance. Even marathon runners who run 18 miles a day know that they can not abruptly increase the distance to 36 miles without risking debilitating fatigue and stress fractures. They slowly and gradually increase the distance to improve their cardiovascular endurance. All athletes should follow their example.

Sample cardiovascular endurance conditioning exercises are presented on page 72.

Muscular Endurance

Muscular endurance enables an athlete to perform muscle movements over and over again without suffering debilitating fatigue. Sometimes muscular endurance is confused with muscular strength and so athletes condition for strength and ignore the need for endurance. The fact is, although muscular endurance and muscle strength work together to help the body perform at optimal levels, they are different muscle functions; they work off different systems of energy, and they need different kinds of conditioning.

For example, if your children can do push-ups, they have the necessary muscle strength to perform the feat, but they may not have the endurance to do ten in a row. In the same way, a tennis player with the strength to hit a return volley to the far corner of the court needs strength plus muscular endurance to make the same shot after an hour of play. And the basketball player who has the strength to sink a basketball from the foul line needs more than just strength to practice the shot twenty times; he or she also needs muscular endurance.

Slow-twitch Muscle Fibers

A person's ultimate capacity for muscular endurance is genetically determined by two factors. First, to sustain repeated movements, the muscles need a continuous and sufficient supply of oxygen. As explained earlier, available oxygen supply (aerobic capacity) varies from individual to individual. Secondly, just as the number of fast-twitch fibers in each muscle determines speed, the slow-twitch variety determines muscular endurance. Slow-twitch fibers work during slow-paced muscle contractions. Although they generate a small amount of force and can't produce the powerful sprint like fast-twitch fibers can, they do not tire quickly. Athletes with a high percentage of them are "natural" endurance athletes and are often among the world-class long-distance runners, skiers, swimmers, and cyclists. As helpful as these fibers are in supporting their chosen sport, it's interesting to note that because these athletes have a higher percentage of slow-twitch fibers, they may drop from exhaustion after sprinting 50 yards at a family picnic.

Training

Even though the maximum degree of muscular endurance is determined by nature, conditioning can certainly improve your athlete's ability to compete without fatigue. This is because in the majority of cases, even "in shape" athletes are far below their maximum endurance level. The previous section explained how aerobic training can give the respiratory, circulatory, and muscular systems the boost needed to improve oxygen intake, transport, and utilization. In addition to enhancing cardiovascular endurance, this kind of training can also build muscular endurance.

Despite the fact that athletes can not increase the number of slow-twitch fibers in their bodies, they can improve the way the available ones work. Many professional athletic trainers believe that the best way to improve muscular endurance is to imitate the body movement as it is used in the sport repeatedly. For instance, to gain leg-muscle endurance a basketball player might practice jump shots, or simply the jumping motion, over and over again. For arm-muscle endurance, a tennis player might continuously hit the ball against the wall.

Sample muscular endurance conditioning exercises are presented on page 72.

Muscular Strength

Muscular strength is the maximum force that can be exerted by a group of muscles. Without a doubt, athletes who develop it have an advantage over opponents who do not. Many parents worry, however, that strength training, which often includes weightlifting, may be too strenuous. Pediatricians and orthopedists are often asked, "My child wants to lift weights; is it safe?" The answer to this question depends in part on the athlete's age.

Age Considerations

Medical research has little to say about the risk-benefit aspects of strength training for children before the onset of puberty. But even without long-term studies or established guidelines, physicians and athletic trainers generally agree that such training for some prepubescent athletes, while possible, should be approached with caution.

The prepubescent child is a male or female, up to 15 or 16 years of age, who has not yet developed secondary sex characteristics such as pubic hair, deepening of voice in boys, and breast development in girls.

In the realm of strength training, these children can be divided into two groups:

1. Children ages 10 and under

   There is no documented proof that strength training has any long-lasting effects on children in this age group. In these athletes, signs of increasing strength will appear as the natural outcome of growth and development—not from training.

2. Children between the ages of 11 and puberty

   Under certain conditions, these athletes may safely begin to experiment with strength training. Training may begin on the condition that the younger child has the emotional maturity to listen to, learn from, and follow without exception the directions of the training coach. Also, the youth must work with a supervisor who has strength-training knowledge, can demonstrate proper technique, and knows the physical limitations of prepubescent athletes.

Because growth spurts (which commonly occur in prepubescent children) will cause muscle tension and inflexibility, it is unwise for athletes in this age group to lift weights at or near their maximum capability; this can cause a muscle tear (page 265) or an avulsion fracture (page 236). Also, the National Strength and Conditioning Association (NSCA) believes that, in addition to strength training, 50 to 80 percent of the prepubescent athlete's training must include a variety of exercises that enhance the other components of athletic performance, such as flexibility, speed, agility, cardiovascular endurance and muscular endurance.[3]

High school athletes who have reached puberty have the most to gain from strength training. In fact, because it's now in vogue, these athletes probably need this kind of conditioning to remain competitive. However, they also need to approach strength training cautiously and slowly, which means learning proper training form, body alignment, and technique. This knowledge, along with appropriate supervision and repetitive practice based on progressive overload, will greatly reduce any risk involved in strength training and enhance its benefits.

Girls vs. Boys

Girls and boys do not naturally develop the same degree of muscular strength. Generally, boys display greater strength at every age without training or conditioning. They have 30 to 50 percent more natural arm strength, yet possess equal capacity in their legs. It's not known if this discrepancy is genetically determined or if it is the result of social conditioning.

In any event strength training can improve the athletic performance of both boys and girls if they set realistic goals. Pre-teen boys, for example, should clearly understand that, through conditioning, they may gain muscular strength, but they will not build muscle bulk. Muscles can not enlarge beyond normal growth size without the male sex hormone, testosterone. Boys do not produce this until the onset of puberty. If, after a few weeks of strength training, you find your young boy flexing in front of the mirror looking for bulging muscles, you'll know he does not understand how the workouts affect his muscles.

High school boys past the age of puberty can strengthen *and* build muscle mass. They still need to realize, however, that increased muscle size comes about over a long period of time and only with consistent training. The vast majority of boys will never build Mr. Universe-type muscles. Parents and coaches can help high school boys set realistic and beneficial strength-training goals.

Girls too need to know what strength training can and can not do for and to their bodies. Some worry that with strength training, they'll look muscle-bound. Others are attracted to the growing trend of body-building for women and want to develop bulging muscles. Both groups of girls need to know that, although females can tone, firm, and strengthen muscles, they can not create substantial muscle mass. Like prepubescent boys, they lack the male hormone that is needed to create bulk. Women who are committed to body-building must take anabolic steroids, a synthetic form of testosterone, to enlarge their muscles. The dangers of anabolic steroids for both girls and boys are discussed in detail in Chapter Five. For now, suffice it to say, under no circumstances should your athletes take anabolic steroids to enhance their athletic performance.

Benefits

Experts once believed that strength training was counter-productive for athletes. They feared that additional muscle mass would make the athlete "muscle-bound" and therefore reduce flexibility, speed, and ease of motion. Recent research has found, however, that just the opposite is true: proper strength training improves muscular strength and can actually increase flexibility, enhance speed by improving the anaerobic bursts in fast-twitch fibers, and add to the fluidity and range of body movement. Also, since strong athletes are usually well trained, they reduce both risk of injury and injury recovery time.

Although muscular strength is always an asset, some sports need it more than others. As you can see on Chart 3.1 (page 47), football linemen and gymnasts need exceptional strength, while tennis players, cross-country skiers, and distance runners need it the least. If your child is putting together a fitness program for a particular sport, be sure to ask the coach if strength training will be beneficial and then check the conditioning information on that sport in Part II of this book.

Strength Training or Weightlifting?

Before giving your okay to strength training, you should first know that there is a difference between that and weightlifting. Weightlifting is a competitive sport in which participants strive to lift the maximum weight possible. Strength training, on the other hand, utilizes free weights, machines, and the athlete's own body weight to increase the ability to exert force. This is done through very gradual overload and progression and always at a point below maximum capability. Strength training is generally a safe and beneficial part of a conditioning program; weightlifting is not.

The two are quickly distinguished from each other in the first few seconds of participation. If your athlete is given a free weight that he or she can not easily lift in repetition more than five to eight times, the training emphasizes weightlifting, not strength training. If, on the other hand, he or she begins with a weight that can be lifted at least five to eight times with fluidity in both the up and down flexing movements, the program focuses on strength training as it should.

Three Methods of Strength Training

There are three popular methods of strength training: isometric, isotonic, and isokinetic. All three are safe and effective methods of building muscular strength and so the choice of method most often depends on available facilities and equipment.

Isometric

The isometric method uses exercises in which one pushes or pulls against an immovable object, or in which one set of muscles pulls against another. Hold on to the seat of your chair; now try to lift it off the ground. The muscle tension you feel in your arms is the result of isometric training. These kinds of exercises strengthen muscles and joints by tensing.

In addition to providing for general strength gain, isometrics are an excellent way to rehabilitate injuries. Joints that would be unduly strained with other kinds of exercise can instead be strengthened progressively, and muscles that would weaken from inactivity inside a cast can also be exercised with this tense/relax/repeat type of exercise program.

Isometric strength training is easy, inexpensive, and effective. It does not require any special equipment; it uses only the muscles of the body and sometimes an immovable object such as the wall. It can be performed almost anywhere at anytime—even in the family room while watching TV—and can not strain the muscles or cause muscle tears or avulsion fractures.

However, isometrics alone can not give maximum strength benefits. They should be combined with isotonic and isokinetic exercises for full benefit of training.

Isotonic

The isotonic method of strength training encompasses any activity in which muscles move a weighted object. Push-ups and sit-ups are isotonic exercises that use the body as weight. Lifting barbells and dumbbells use free weights. Most isotonic strength training programs use a combination of both body and free weight exercises.

Isotonics use repetition to build muscular strength. The number of times an athlete can lift a given weight determines the outcome in gained strength. The American Academy of Orthopedic Surgeons believes that young athletes can best enhance their strength by doing eight to ten repetitions of a weight that is 60 to 70 percent of what they can maximally lift. For example, if they can lift a maximum of 100 pounds on a bench press, they should work out with a 60 to 70 pound weight for eight to ten repetitions. When they can increase the reps to twelve and maintain the same level of ease of exercise and fluidity of motion before feeling fatigued, they can move up to a heavier weight.

Isotonics are popular strength-gain exercises. Most high school, local, and home gymnasiums are equipped with the relatively inexpensive free weights, and so the equipment is the kind most readily available. But even athletes who do not have access to these weights can still use the isotonic method by using their own body weight to exert force with exercises like push-ups, sit-ups, and pull-ups.

The only disadvantage of the isotonic method is the fact that it must be closely supervised. The amount of weight an athlete lifts should be determined by someone trained to judge capability. The lifting session itself must be monitored to ensure that athletes are performing the lifts properly, that they are not overworking their muscles and are protected from injury by trained spotters.

Isokinetics

The isokinetic method of strength training uses rather sophisticated machines such as the Cybex, Kin-Com, and Biodex to move the muscles against an even pressure. Research indicates that, in general, isokinetic exercise best strengthens muscles for sports activity—but unfortunately the machines are quite expensive and not readily available to youth athletes.

A popular exercise machine is the Nautilus. It is actually a cross between isotonic and isokinetic methods. The machine strengthens muscles with weights as well as with a system of pulley and lever actions. These machines are usually more readily available and are excellent for working on specific body parts.

Whether your children use isotonic or isokinetic, or a combination of the two, they should remember that strength training works on the principles of adaption, overload, and progression.

Strength Training Guidelines

Athletes over the age of ten who want to improve muscular strength can do it safely and effectively. They need both close supervision by a trained instructor, however, and a set of realistic goals. They should balance their training regime with other kinds of body conditioning. And they need to know HOW to train and how NOT to train to avoid injury. The list of Don'ts on the following page is adapted from the book *Joe Weider's Weight Training for Sports*. If you can ensure that your young athlete follows these guidelines, his or her strength training experience will be a positive and productive one.

Over-Training

The principle rule of sports conditioning is, "Train, don't strain." Over-training defeats the purpose of conditioning because instead of becoming tougher from long, tortuous practices and workouts, kids become more prone to injury. As your young athlete begins his or her sports program, watch for these signs of over-training:

- feelings of extreme tiredness and listlessness during workouts
- chronic fatigue
- prolonged soreness in the joints and tendons
- insomnia
- irritability
- decreased interest in sports-play
- reduced speed, strength, and endurance
- slower reflexes

These symptoms will appear at any level of play when youngsters are pushed beyond their physical capabilities. If you notice signs of over-training, it's important to help the athlete recover before the fatigued body becomes injured. You can do this by:

- allowing one to two days off from training
- having your child engage in relaxing activities such as rec-

THE DON'TS OF
WEIGHT TRAINING

- Don't lift weights before reading about weight training or getting advice from a competent coach. Train smart for the best progress.
- Don't ever lift heavier weights than your weight training program calls for. Doing maximum lifts just to show how strong you are can be dangerous. It is not helpful in preparing you for your sport and, in fact, can be detrimental to your training program.
- Don't train with weights before skill training. Fatigue will hamper your efforts at acquiring skill. Do weight training exercises after your skill training, or train on days when no skill practice is taking place.
- Don't train with weights before running. Tired leg muscles from squats, or other leg exercises, means that your hip and knee joints are unable to offer you the support you need. Running causes a great deal of jarring of these joints. Injury can result.
- Don't forget to use safety equipment such as locking collars on weights and proper training attire. Be sure there is plenty of room around you when exercising to ensure accident-free training. Be sure the equipment you are using is in good condition. A simple inspection of the free weights or exercise machines beforehand is a wise precaution.
- Don't leave weights scattered on the floor or leaning against other equipment. The single biggest cause of gym injuries is due to not putting weights back on their storage racks. Keep a neat, tidy gym to avoid accidents.
- Don't try to unload a bar one end at a time. Taking weight plates off the bar on one side only causes the other side to become unbalanced and fall from the rack, sometimes with great speed and force. Be safe and unload plates from the bar by alternating from one end to the other.
- Don't drop weights to the floor. Dropping weights causes equipment damage, floor damage, and can be dangerous.
- Don't train without a proper sweatshirt on. Your perspiration makes your body very slippery and may cause you to lose your balance, or slide while you are lying on your back on a bench, thus losing control of the weight you are lifting. When you place the bar on your shoulders a slight slip due to perspiration can cause a pulled muscle, or worse while you try to regain control of the weight. Last, it's a courtesy to your fellow trainer; wet, slippery benches are unpleasant to use.
- Don't neglect your warm-up and flexibility exercises. Weight training is stressful to your muscles. You should not forget to stretch them first and ensure that each muscle is properly warmed up before lifting begins.
- Don't forget to keep a training log (p. 219). Your continued progress depends upon keeping a record of each training session and the weights lifted. Include the amounts of reps-sets, your body measurements, arms, legs, waist, chest, and neck circumference. Keeping such records, along with your body weight over the weeks and months of training, enables you to follow your own progress closely. You can see where adjustments are necessary. You can control your progress.
- Don't neglect any part of your body. Your training program should emphasize every major muscle. This is necessary to build a solid foundation for years of sports participation. Sometimes beginners in weight training only do arm and chest exercises. These show up muscle development quicker and seem to be more fun to do, but such an unbalanced program will just result in an unbalanced body. Your whole body is equally important.
- Don't miss workouts. A serious athlete sets a program, makes a commitment, and then sticks to it. If your training is to work, it must be done regularly.
- Don't lift weights alone when you get into training with heavier weights. Accidents can be avoided when a training partner is available to help. However, for the first six months you will not be working with such heavy weights that a partner is necessary. But it is more fun to train with a friend than alone and, if you can get into the routine of working with a partner, it will come naturally later on when you progress to heavier weights and will need some help.

reational play (active rest), warm baths, and sore muscle massage
- checking the athlete's diet for proper nutritional intake

When your athlete returns to sports practice, you should talk to the coaches about the symptoms you've observed. Expressing your concerns about over-training will alert the coaches to the possibility of practice routines that are too strenuous. This kind of open dialogue will also caution the coaches to watch for any further problems in this area. Then be sure to carefully monitor your child's eating and sleeping habits (see Chapter Two) to ensure that the body has what it needs to recover from the daily training regime.

Sample Conditioning Exercises

Flexibility

1. Neck:
   - With hands on hips, slowly rotate neck in full circle. Hold the stretch where neck feels tight.
   Repeat 10 times in both directions.
2. Shoulders:
   - In standing position with arms parallel to the floor, rotate arms in a full circle.
   Repeat 10 times in both directions.
   - In a standing position with knees slightly bent, gently pull elbow behind head as you bend from your hips to the side. Hold for 10 seconds. Repeat on other side.
   - In a standing position, grab a towel near both ends so you can move it with straight arms up and over your head and down behind your back. Do not strain or force. Hold mild stretch for 10 to 20 seconds.
3. Tricep/Shoulders:
   - In a standing position with your arms overhead, hold

the elbow of one arm with the hand of the other. Slowly pull your elbow behind your head.

4. Side:
   - In a standing position with arms overhead, bend to the side. When bending to the left, clasp your right wrist with your left hand and pull down slowly. Reverse for the right side.

5. Hamstring:
   - In a standing position, put your feet shoulder-width apart and pointed straight ahead. Slowly bend forward from the hips, keeping your knees slightly bent. Let your neck and arms relax. Stretch to the point where you feel slight stretch in the back of your legs. Hold for 15 to 25 seconds. Keep your knees slightly bent when returning to a standing position.
   - While standing, raise one leg to a comfortable level and place it on a secure support. Look straight ahead and bend forward at your waist. Hold and relax. Repeat with the other leg.

6. Hamstring, Lower Back, and Side:
   - Stand upright with feet together. Bend at the waist. Keep knees locked and grab your ankles. Slowly pull your chest down to your knees.
   - Stand with your feet apart. Turn your right foot out to the right and bring your chest down to the right knee. Do the same with the left.
   - In the sitting position, extend legs together out in front of your body. Grab your ankles and try to put your nose on your knees. Hold that position for ten seconds.

7. Lower Back:
   - Lie on your back. Bring your knees up to your chest. Wrap your arms around your knees and roll up in a ball.

8. Lower Back and Hips:
   - Lie on your back. Bring your legs over your head and touch your toes to the ground while keeping your knees

straight. Keep your hands on your hips or flat on the ground to maintain balance.

9. Groin and Hip:
   - While standing, place the ball of your foot on a secure raised support. Keep the other leg straight. Bend the raised knee as you move your hips forward. Hold for 30 seconds. Repeat with other leg.

10. Groin:
    - While seated on the floor, pull the soles of your feet together with your hands and elbows inside of the knee. Push out with the elbows and try to touch the outside of your knee and leg to the ground. Repeat 2 times.
    - While sitting, put the soles of your feet together and hold on to your toes. Gently pull your body forward, bending from the hips, until you feel a stretch in the groin area. Hold for 40 seconds.

11. Quadriceps:
    - While lying face down on your stomach, bring your heels up toward your back and reach back with your hands to grab your ankles. Pull on your ankles and as you arch your back, bring your eyes to the sky.

12. Calf and Achilles Tendon:
    - Face a wall with the feet spread approximately three feet from the baseboard. Lean into the wall and use the arms to lower the body towards the wall until the calf muscle is taut. Hold that position for ten seconds.
    - Stand about 2 feet away from a wall. Leaning your forearms on the wall, rest your head on your hands. Bend one leg with the other one straight behind. Slowly move your hips forward, keeping your lower back flat and your heel on the ground. Hold for 30 seconds. Repeat with the other leg.

13. Hips:
    - Sit down with one leg in a semi-bent position behind the body and a bit off to the side. Lean backward to

stretch the front thighs. Hold for five to ten seconds. Repeat with other leg.
- In a half-kneeling position, move one leg forward until the knee is directly over the ankle; the other knee should be resting on the floor. Lower the hip to create an easy stretch. Hold for 30 seconds. Repeat on other side.

14. Ankle and Heel Cord:
- Kneel on the floor. Bring one foot up to sit flat, even with the opposite knee. Then sit back as far as you can on your back foot. Next, lean forward with your shoulder against the knee. As you lean forward try to keep the sole of your foot flat. Hold this position for ten seconds.

15. Chest and Shoulder:
- Stretch your arms up over your head. Lock your fingers together. Try to drop your arms down behind your back as far as you can. You may have to unclasp your hands and move your arms apart when you first try this stretch.

16. Shoulder and Arm:
- In a standing position with arms straight, interlock your fingers behind your back. Slowly turn your elbows inward while straightening your arms; then lift your arms up until you feel a stretch in the shoulder and chest. Hold for 10 seconds.

17. Forearm and Wrist:
- Kneel down. Place your palms flat on the floor with your fingers pointing back toward your knees. Lean slightly forward and hold for five seconds.

18. Rotator Cuff and Front Shoulder:
- Stand sideways next to a wall. Put your arm up and straight at shoulder length and put your palm flat against

the wall. As you press your weight against the wall, turn your body away from the wall slightly.

Agility

1. Bounding:
   - Do a series of 20 fast, standing, two-legged long jumps.
2. Jumprope Drills:
   - Begin rope jumping at an easy pace with both feet together. Jump on one foot at a time and move on to alternate feet. Then try kicking your feet in and out while jumping and add variation by bringing your knees up high. Finally, try each rope jumping style while criss-crossing your arms.

     When you jump rope, make sure you do it correctly. The rope should be ⅜ of an inch thick and should fit your body size—the ends should just reach your armpits when you stand on the middle of the rope. To execute the exercise properly, lower your body by bending your knees, and push off from your toes by straightening your knees. Don't jump more than one inch off the ground, and be sure to land on the balls of your feet.
3. Side Running:
   - Run sideways while criss-crossing your feet. Make your steps quick and small.
4. Bench Jumps:
   - Jump back and forth sideways over a narrow bench approximately 18 inches high for 30 seconds.

Speed

1. Repeat Intervals:
   - Run continuously for one-quarter to one-half a mile. During this run, vary the speed in one of two ways:
   - a. Run at top speed for 100 yards, and then jog slowly for 100 yards. Repeat until the body becomes fatigued.

    b. Run at top speed for as long as possible. Then jog slowly until you recover enough energy to sprint out at top speed again. Again, reduce speed when you tire and sprint out when you can.
2. Acceleration Sprints:
- Running at full speed for a short distance a number of times builds endurance and fast-twitch fibers.

Cardiovascular Endurance

1. Distance Running:
- At a slow pace, run as far as you can. Push yourself to run just a bit past your initial point of tiredness. Increase the distance with each conditioning session.
2. Bicycling:
- Long-distance bicycling or stationary bicycling can also build endurance. This is a good off-season exercise for all sports.
3. Repeat Intervals:
- See Speed Exercise #1 above.

Muscular Endurance

1. Backward Sprints:
- Sprint 10 yards backwards; turn around and sprint back to the starting line. Then sprint 20 yards backwards; turn around and sprint those 20 yards back to the starting line. Sprint 30 yards backwards; turn around and sprint those 30 yards back to the starting line. This drill is especially helpful to build endurance in the leg muscles.
2. Bike Riding:
- Bicycle riding will build endurance in the leg and back muscles.

Muscular Strength

1. Abdominals
Crunches:

- Lie on the floor with your feet resting up on the bench. Clasp your fingers behind your head. Then in a sit-up fashion, try to touch your ribs to your hips by squeezing your abdomen together.

Dumbbell Sidebend:
- Hold only one dumbbell in one hand at your side. Raise your other arm up behind your head as you bend toward the side with the weight. Make sure to hold a weight that is heavy enough to give you a full stretch.

2. Arms

Reverse Curl:
- Hold dumbbells at your sides with palms facing in. Keeping your elbow in close to your body, bend the elbow to raise the weight up to shoulder level with palm facing inward toward the body. Return to the resting position. Repeat with opposite arm.

French Press:
- Stand with your feet spread approximately two feet apart. Hold the dumbbell at your side. Raise the weight to a straight-arm position overhead then bend your elbow to bring the weight down behind your head. Straighten your elbow to return the weight to a straight arm position, then return to the resting position. Repeat with opposite arm.

3. Back

Chin-ups:
- Standard chin-ups are an excellent exercise for strengthening back muscles.

Hyperextensions:
- Lie face down on a table with your stomach at the edge. Make sure your feet are secured or have someone hold them. Clasp your hands around the back of your head. Then slowly bend at the waist to lower your upper body down toward the floor. Then return back up to the starting position. Do not force the extension beyond a

parallel position because this can be injurious to the spine.

4. Calf
   Calf Raises:
   - Rest bar weights behind your head on your shoulders. With feet slightly apart, push up to stand on your toes. Hold. And return to resting position.

5. Chest
   Dumbbell Flye:
   - Lie on your back on the bench. Holding lightweight dumbbells in both hands, stretch your arms out straight. Lift the weights directly overhead until your hands meet. Slowly return to the starting position.
   Bench:
   - Lie on your back on the bench. Bring the bar down just below the pectorals and touch the chest lightly. Then extend the arms fully to the straight-arm position.

6. Groin
   Leg Adductor and Abductor Lifts:
   - These exercises are best done with a cable attachment hooked to the ankle or knee. Balance yourself by holding on to the wall or nearby support. With straight leg, lift the leg back and up. Then return to resting position. After a series of lifts, repeat the exercise with the opposite leg. Also, turn and lift the straight leg out to the side and up as far as you are able. Return the leg to the resting position. After a series of these lifts, repeat the exercise with the opposite leg.

7. Hips
   Roman Chair Sit-ups:
   - Secure your feet on the lower bar of the Roman chair. Placing your hands on your abdomen, lean back as far as you can comfortably go and then return to a sitting position.

8. Knee
   Leg Extension:
   - Sit at the end of the bench holding on to the sides. Tuck your feet under the roll-bar weights. Lift your legs until they are parallel with the rest of your lower body, then lower them back down. Use slow controlled movements rather than quick explosive ones.

9. Legs
   Squats:
   - Set the bar on the back of your shoulders and on top of the scapula. With your feet at shoulder width, squat to a 75-degree angle, then stand erect.
   Leg Press:
   - On a bench inclined at 45 degrees, with knees bent, set both feet against a weight and push forward and return to starting position. If you place your feet high on the weight, you'll work the gluteus and hamstring muscles. With the feet placed lower you'll develop the quadriceps.

10. Shoulders
    Front Dumbbell Press:
    - From a sitting position, hold a lightweight dumbbell in each hand at shoulder level. Raise the weights overhead until your arms are straight. Bend elbows and bring the weights back down to shoulder level.
    Lateral Raise:
    - Holding a dumbbell in each hand with arms at your side, bring your arms slightly forward and bend your elbows. Then raise the arms straight up and out to the side. Stop when your arms are slightly past your shoulders. Slowly return your arms to the resting position.
    Cleans:
    - Stand directly over the bar with your feet shoulder-width apart. Grasp the bar and lift it straight up, keeping it as close to your body as possible. At waist level, snap the bar up to the chest by dropping the elbows and

extending the mid-section in a forward thrust. Keep your back straight.

11. Wrist
    Wrist Curls:
    • Using an E-Z curl bar, rest your forearms on the pad and grab the bar with both hands from underneath. Using wrist action only, lift the bar up and return it back to its place.

12. Hands
    Athletes can strengthen the muscles in their hands by climbing ropes, doing fingertip push-ups, and catching and passing a medicine ball.

13. Ankle
    Ankle Extensor Lift:
    • Lying in a face-down position, extend arms above the head with palms down. Bend the knee at a right angle with the lower leg vertical to the table. Move the raised foot into a position of maximal stretch with the toes reaching toward the front of the leg. Then lift the foot upward as far as possible and lower slowly to the starting position. Throughout the movement, the leg must remain still. For variation, the foot can be lifted upward, backward, and outward. The exercise can also be performed with the knees straight, with the legs extended beyond the edge of the table.

4

■ ■ ■ ■ ■

The Pre-Season Medical Exam

A general objective of pre-season medical exams is to identify conditions that might interfere with safe participation in physical activities. Therefore, a medical examination prior to participation in a sports program should be a vital component of your plan to keep your young athlete healthy. Because there are no national standards for sports examinations, however, each athletic organization is free to develop a system of pre-season physicals that best meets the program's personal objectives as well as its financial, environmental, and personnel resources. That's why you need to monitor how the examinations are given, exactly what the physical is expected to accomplish, and if it is appropriate for your young athlete's special needs in his or her chosen sport.

The most neglected group of athletes, in regard to pre-season physicals, is the prepubescent child (ages 6–10). Most leagues on this level of play (excluding most organized football leagues) do not require any type of pre-season medical examination. The athletes join the team, play the season, and everyone hopes for the best. The fact that young players might not be required to have a pre-season check-up does not mean that there is no reason for one. At this age athletes may manifest clinical congenital abnormalities such as heart defects that were not previously diagnosed. If your children intend to play on a sports team that does not offer or require pre-season physicals, be sure to take them to your family doctor for a physical that is thorough and sports specific as explained in this chapter.

Older youth-league players (ages 11–15) and high school athletes are usually required to undergo some type of pre-season evaluation before they are given clearance to participate on an athletic team. Because these athletes are prone to rapid body growth that causes changes in the musculo-skeletal system, and are experiencing physical, psychological, and sexual maturation changes that can affect their ability to play organized sports safely, it is imperative that you oversee the kind of medical evaluation they receive.

Types of Pre-Season Medical Exams

League rules often require sports participants to have pre-season physicals; sometimes these exams are provided by the sports association or school; other times, athletes must make their own arrangements for these physicals. The kind of examination given to the athlete often determines the quality and thoroughness you can expect. Generally, physical exams are given in one of the following three ways.

Locker Room Physicals

Locker room physicals are the least desirable kind of pre-season examination. They tend to be noisy, hurried, and incomplete. A pre-season physical recently administered at a small town high school illustrates the drawbacks of this method. All students who wished to participate in a fall or winter sport (all volleyball, football, basketball, field hockey, soccer, and tennis players, along with wrestlers, gymnasts, and swimmers) were told to meet in the gymnasium on Saturday morning. Along with approximately 300 other young athletes, a promising young gymnast named Jeni arrived for her physical, which was to be administered by a local family practitioner. While Jeni and her teammates waited their turn, they were given a medical history checklist to complete. Jeni noted on the checklist that she had had a previous shoulder injury but did not mention her recent hospitalization for weight loss and fatigue brought on by anorexia nervosa.

When it was Jeni's turn for the physical, the doctor glanced over her medical history form, then checked her pulse rate, peered into her mouth and eyes, and used a stethoscope to listen to her heart. Then, without a word, he signed the form allowing her to participate in the sports program even though without pre-season conditioning, Jeni's shoulder problem will cause her continued pain throughout the season, and her frail body condition was an indication that she needed a follow-up program to monitor her body weight.

This most common example of an assembly-line physical will fulfill the school's insurance requirements and will assess the general superficial health of the athletes. But it is condemned by both the American Academy of Pediatrics and experts in the field of sports medicine because it will do very little to disclose sport specific areas of weakness or personal problems that might put the athlete at risk for injury.[1]

Station Technique

The station-technique method of administering pre-season medical examinations can be an efficient and cost-effective, as well as thorough, method of providing physicals to a large number of athletes over a short period of time. This approach utilizes a primary-care physician along with volunteers from the school system including school nurses, athletic trainers, coaches, and interested teachers and administrators.

The examination area is divided into examination stations.

The largest room accommodates all the athletes and various examination stations. There are also quiet, screened-off office areas close to this large room. The American Academy of Pediatrics recommends the following station organization:

Station 1—Individual History
Station 2—Blood Pressure
Station 3—Vision
Station 4—Skin, Mouth, Eyes
Station 5—Chest
Station 6—Lymphatics, Abdomen, Genitalia
Station 7—Orthopedic Exam
Station 8—Review and Final Assessment[2]

Trained school personnel (coaches, nurses, trainers, and teachers) conduct examinations at stations 1, 2, 3, and 4, while physicians are utilized in the remaining stations.

Individual Examination

An individual examination is performed in the office of the athlete's own doctor. If group examination is not offered by the sports program, all athletes must have an individual exam to ensure safe participation. Even if group examinations are offered by the athletic program, you might still arrange for an individual exam if the locker room method is your only other option, or if your athlete has past injuries or chronic health problems that deserve special attention.

Personal exams have advantages over group exams. 1) The physician already knows the athlete's past medical history. 2) When the doctor and athlete have an established relationship, the youth is more likely to discuss sensitive issues such as drug use, eating habits, sex, physical maturation, and development. 3) There is better continuity of care, especially if the athlete has been previously injured. 4) If the examination uncovers reason for further specialized consultation, arrangements can be made quickly and follow-up care is more complete.

The individual exam does pose several disadvantages for the young athlete. These include a lack of consistency among physicians, leading to inconsistency in judgments concerning qualification, disqualification and referral; lack of familiarity with the demands of specific sports that leads to judgments being either too conservative or too liberal, causing unfairness to the athlete; and the process is not cost-effective and may discourage parents from obtaining the medical exam the athlete needs.[3]

If you have the opportunity to choose between group examinations and individual ones, you should weigh the advantages and disadvantages of each and choose what you feel is best for your young athlete.

The Pre-Season Medical Exam

No matter which type of medical examination you use to assess your athlete's risk of injury, you should look for certain features. These include the following:

Thoroughness

A sports physical should not be viewed as "just a check-up." It should be thorough, complete, and appropriate to the athlete's chosen sport. It should include an evaluation of the following areas:

Individual History

The physician should pay particular attention to the details stated on the individual history form. The objective of this information is to identify risk factors that may predispose an athlete to harm or injury but that may not be detected in the physical exam. These factors include past problems with blood pressure or heart disease, dizziness, fainting during exercise, convulsions or frequent headaches, concussions, joint problems, or missing organs.

Height and Weight

Height and weight measurements should be recorded. This information may alert the physician to eating disorders, steroid use, or late maturation.

Vital Signs

Pulse rate and blood pressure should be taken and recorded. Blood pressure values indicating a need for further evaluation are:

6 to 11 years: > 130/75 mm Hg

12 years and older > 140/85 mm Hg

Pulse rate should range between 55 and 75 and should always be compared with rates taken during previous examinations.

Vision

The vision of all athletes should be tested as part of the pre-season health evaluation. If the vision in either eye is worse than 20/40 with eyeglasses, the athlete should be examined by an ophthalmologist before he or she is given clearance for sports participation.

If your athlete wears eyeglasses you should make sure that the type of lens and frame are safe for sports play. Streetwear glasses should not be used in any sport that poses the potential for eye contact with an object or opponent. Ask your ophthalmologist to recommend one of the following three kinds of protective eyewear:

Class I: A protector with the lens and frame frontpiece molded as one unit.

Class II: A protector with a lens mounted in a frame. Both industrial-safety eyeglasses and specifically designed sports frame/lens combinations are available.

Class III: A protector without a lens, which may be used

alone to protect the eye area, or may be used over the athlete's eyeglasses.

If your young athlete has severely impaired vision or blindness in one eye, you should consult with your ophthalmologist before even considering sports play. Not only might this visual handicap increase the athlete's risk of injury in certain sports, but injury to the functioning eye might alter the child's quality of life.

Skin

The skin is the largest organ of the body. It should be examined closely during the pre-season physical. Warts, blisters, calluses, abrasions, and athlete's foot should be noted by the physician so that treatment, care, and preventive strategies can be discussed with the athlete.

Some skin problems may temporarily disqualify the athlete from contact or swimming sport participation until proper treatment is prescribed. Disqualifying infections include impetigo and herpes simplex (commonly called cold sores or fever blisters); infestations of scabietic mites and crab lice might also keep an athlete from active participation.

Heart

All pre-season physicals must include an exam for cardiovascular abnormalities. Excluding trauma, sudden death in athletes is almost always related to cardiovascular problems.[4] Yet it has never been proven that a normal heart has died under exercise conditions.[5] Therefore it is the aim of the pre-season physical to detect cardiac abnormalities before the heart is overly stressed by physical activity.

Information on the individual history form that indicates the athlete has suffered fainting spells during or after exercise and/or has a family history of early deaths (under age 50) should alert the physician to the need for further cardiac evaluation. Participation clearance should also be withheld pending further evaluation if the physical exam finds pulse discrepancy, murmers, abnormal rhythm, arrhythmias, forced expiratory maneuver, or evidence of latent bronchospasm. Specialized cardiac consultation for athletes with these conditions is recommended to protect them against cardiac-related injury and death. After further evaluation, however, most often children who show signs of these symptoms, and even those with mild heart defects, are able to play and benefit from the sport of their choice.

Abdomen

The child's abdomen should be examined as he or she lies flat on a table. The physician will check for any enlargement of abdominal organs.

Genitalia

A pelvic exam is not necessary for a female athlete unless a question about menstrual abnormalities arises from information offered on the individual history form. The male genitalia should be examined for absent or undescended testicles which, although not a cause for automatic disqualification, do warrant further discussion with the boy's parents to explain the danger of risking injury to the genital area and to recommend the use of a protective cup. Although the physician may routinely check for hernias, it is not necessary since disqualifying hernias will become evident when the athlete complains of pain.

Maturation

The physician should note the breast development and pubic hair distribution of girls, and the genitalia development and pubic hair distribution of boys. This information will enable the physician to determine the athlete's level of physical maturity. Competition between late and early maturers (especially in contact sports) increases the chance of sustaining a sports-related injury by allowing unfair competition between athletes who differ greatly in strength, agility, coordination, and endurance. A maturity lag is not a cause for disqualification, but it is reason for the physician to recommend that the athlete consider delaying his or her participation in a contact sport and consider a non-contact activity.

Musculoskeletal System

Careful attention must be given to the athlete's growing musculoskeletal system. The physician should test for a full range of motion in all the major joints (these include the spine, wrist, knee, elbow, shoulder, hip, foot, and ankle), and for strength in the major muscle groups. He or she should also look for abnormal foot postures that may require the athlete to wear an orthotic device to prevent pain and injury while running. At this time the physician may also be able to diagnose deterioration of a compromised limb that causes chronic pain. He or she may also note if the pain is caused by some other previously asymptomatic condition of childhood or adolescence. Chronic foot pain in a soccer player, for example, may not be an overuse injury as initially diagnosed if there is a history of inflammatory arthritis or other connective tissue diseases in the family. The following chart lists a commonly used orthopedic screening examination that is designed to reveal previous injuries which have been inadequately rehabilitated and those previously unrecognized orthopedic conditions that might be adversely affected by sports play. This entire exam takes about 90 seconds to administer.

Neurology

As a final indicator of sports readiness, the physician should give a general neurologic exam to check for problems with

CHART 4.1
ORTHOPEDIC SCREENING EXAMINATION°

The orthopedic screening examination requires about 90 seconds. Time studies indicate it is most efficiently done one athlete at a time rather than in small groups. It is designed to reveal previous inadequately rehabilitated injuries or those few previously unrecognized orthopedic conditions that might be adversely affected by participation in a sports activity. Positive findings require a more extensive examination and/or history. A more detailed examination **should not** be attempted at the screening examination.

Athletic Activity (Instructions)	Observation
Stand facing examiner	Acromioclavicular joints; general habitus
Look at ceiling, floor, over both shoulders; touch ears to shoulders	Cervical spine motion
Shrug shoulders (examiner resists)	Trapezius strength
Abduct shoulders 90° (examiner resists at 90°)	Deltoid strength
Full external rotation of arms	Shoulder motion
Flex and extend elbows	Elbow motion
Arms at sides, elbows 90° flexed; pronate and supinate wrists	Elbow and wrist motion
Spread fingers; make fist	Hand or finger motion and deformities
Tighten (contact) quadriceps; relax quadriceps	Symmetry and knee effusion; ankle effusion
"Duck walk" four steps (away from examiner with buttocks on heels)	Hip, knee, and ankle motion
Back to examiner	Shoulder symmetry; scoliosis
Knees straight, touch toes	Scoliosis, hip motion, hamstring tightness
Raise up on toes, raise heels	Calf symmetry, leg strength

° May require reflex hammer, tape measure, pin, and examination table.

peripheral nerves, strength, reflexes, balance, and coordination. If a significant weakness in this area is uncovered, the young athlete should be examined by a neurologist before being cleared for sports participation. Neurological problems can indicate an underlying illness or injury which may seriously jeopardize the child's health.

Laboratory Tests

Laboratory tests are not a necessary part of a pre-season physical. Although a physician may routinely include a urinalysis for protein and glucose as well as blood tests for hemoglobin and hematocrit, the American Academy of Pediatrics has stated, "There is now abundant documentation that the routine urinalysis on healthy, unsymptomatic populations is unrewarding and a cause of unnecessary anxiety." They have further stated, "In today's healthy athletes, these laboratory studies [urinalysis and hemoglobin/hematocrit determination] contribute only added expense and some logistic complications."[6]

It is recommended, however, that black athletes have a blood test for the sickle cell trait. It has been documented that under heat conditions and high altitudes black soldiers with the sickle cell trait have died of exercise deaths.[7]

Body Conditioning

Because the goal of the pre-season medical exam is to find areas of physical weakness which may predispose an athlete to injury, many sports-clinic personnel, trainers, and knowledgeable physicians are now including an evaluation of body conditioning in this initial exam. Athletes are tested for sport-specific flexibility, cardiovascular fitness, muscular strength, and when appropriate, body fat composition. (See Chapter Three for a complete discussion of body conditioning.) The results of these tests are not used to exclude an athlete from participation, but rather to identify areas that need improvement and to give a baseline for a pre-season conditioning program that will enable the athlete to enter the sports season in good shape.

An exam of body condition will also point out overdeveloped dominant extremities. If, for example, a tennis player has exceptionally developed right hand and arm muscles, he or she should be advised to work on strengthening the non-dominant hand to balance the body muscles. This cross-training strengthening will also prevent injury to the weaker muscle group when the athlete switches to another recreational or competitive activity.

Sport Specificity

The pre-season examination should be given by a physician who is knowledgeable in the field of pediatric sports medicine and who is able to give special attention to the anatomical areas that are frequently the site of medical problems in your child's particular sport. (See Chart 4.2.) A pre-season exam for a football player should not be the same as one for a tennis player. And unlike these athletes, weight-matched and endurance sport athletes should be examined and then in addition offered medical and nutritional guidance that will teach them how to obtain optimal weight and body fat levels. Exceptional programs offer athletes pre-training physicals, pre-season physicals, and mid-season reviews to allow for careful monitoring of the athlete's physical condition. This allows the physician to identify low-grade injuries, muscular growth weaknesses, and overuse syndromes in their early stages, and intervene before the condition become debilitating.

Timing

Pre-season sports physicals should be given at a time that is not too close to the beginning of the season and yet not too far away. The medical examination should be far enough away from the beginning of the season to allow an athlete time for consultation with a specialist if recommended, for rehabilitation of correctable problems, for body conditioning when recommended, and for weight adjustment if necessary. The exam should not be so far away from the sport season, however, that the athlete could develop a precluding condition or sustain a disqualifying injury between the time of the

CHART 4.2
SPORT STRESS AREAS

SPORT	STRESSED BODY PARTS
Baseball/Softball	shoulder, elbow, arm, hamstrings, Achilles tendons, hips, lower back
Basketball	ankle, shoulder, upper arms, calves, back, Achilles tendons
Football	all upper and lower extremities and the cervical spine
Gymnastics	all upper and lower extremities and the cervical spine
Ice Hockey	legs, shoulders, rotator cuff, hips
Lacrosse	shoulders, knees, ankles, upper legs, and hands
Long-Distance Running	back, hip, knee, ankle, foot
Skiing	lower extremities
Soccer	hips, pelvis, foot, lower legs, Achilles tendon, neck
Swimming	ears, shoulders, knees, chest, back
Tennis	shoulder, elbow, wrist, Achilles tendons
Volleyball	fingers, ankles, shoulders, knees, legs, hips, upper arms
Wrestling	neck, shoulders, skin, upper legs, hands

physical and the onset of the season. A recommended time-table is 6 to 8 weeks before the season begins.

Frequency

Most athletes do not need a medical examination prior to every new sport season. A complete and thorough exam is recommended every three to four years, which usually co-incides with the beginning of junior high, senior high, and college. During the years in between, athletes should visit their team or family physicians so that they can follow up the rehabilitation of previous injuries, review vital signs, discuss all injuries and illnesses which have occurred since the last exam, note if the athlete is wearing any new appliances such as glasses, contacts, or braces, and offer the athletes an opportunity to discuss personal health concerns.

Final Assessment

The final assessment of an athlete's ability to engage in physical activity should not be a blanket clearance or disqualification. The decision should be made taking into consideration the type of sport the athlete wishes to play and the other options available to the athlete.

The following classification of sports chart is based on each sport's physical requirements, which includes degree of body contact, endurance requirements, and general physical ability needed to participate. The chart classifies sports as contact, limited-contact, non-contact, moderately strenuous, and non-strenuous. The approval or denial of participation for athletes with questionable medical conditions must be made by a physician knowledgeable in the distinctions between these sport categories.

There are no absolutes in the list of disqualifying conditions; each athlete deserves individual evaluation and counseling to guide him or her to an appropriate form of physical exercise. The chart on page 92, "Disqualifying Conditions for Sports Participation," was formulated in 1979 by the American Medical Association. Although the recommendations have not been reviewed in light of recent growing data and medical information, it still serves as a base from which physicians can consider their options. Most commonly these options include:

1. clearance without limitation for the sport and level desired.
2. clearance deferred pending consultation, special treatment, special equipment fitting, or rehabilitation.

CHART 4.3
CLASSIFICATION OF SPORTS

Strenuous			Moderately Strenuous	Nonstrenuous
Contact	Limited Contact	Noncontact		
Football	Basketball	Crew	Badminton	Archery
Ice hockey	Field hockey	Cross	Baseball	Bowling
Lacrosse (boys)	Lacrosse (girls)	country	(limited	Riflery
Rugby	Soccer	Fencing	contact)	
Wrestling	Volleyball	Swimming	Golf	
	Gymnastics	Tennis	Table tennis	
	Skiing	Track and	Curling	
		field		
		Water polo		

3. clearance with limitation to include medical recommendations for another sport.
4. disqualification which implies that the athlete has a condition which precludes him or her from participation in any sport.[8]

If your child's physician should recommend option numbers 3 or 4, you, your child, the doctor, and the coach should discuss the situation to be sure that all factors such as sport type, player position, and available treatment and rehabilitation options have been thoroughly considered. Chapter Eighteen will give you more information about sports participation for children with chronic illness.

CHART 4.4
DISQUALIFYING CONDITIONS FOR SPORTS PARTICIPATION

Conditions	Colli-sion°	Contact†	Non-contact‡	Other§
General				
Acute infections: Respiratory, genitourinary, infectious mononucleosis, hepatitis, active rheumatic fever, active tuberculosis	X	X	X	X
Obvious physical immaturity in comparison with other competitors	X	X		
Hemorrhagic disease: Hemophilia, purpura, and other serious bleeding tendencies	X	X	X	
Diabetes, inadequately controlled	X	X	X	X
Diabetes, controlled	††	††	††	††
Jaundice	X	X	X	X
Eyes				
Absence or loss of function of one eye	X	X		
Respiratory				
Tuberculosis (active or symptomatic)	X	X	X	X
Severe pulmonary insufficiency	X	X	X	X
Cardiovascular				
Mitral stenosis, aortic stenosis, aortic insufficiency, coarctation of aorta, cyanotic heart disease, recent carditis or any etiology	X	X	X	X
Hypertension on organic basis	X	X	X	X
Previous heart surgery for congenital or acquired heart disease	‖	‖	‖	‖
Liver, enlarged	X	X		

° Football, rugby, hockey, lacrosse, and so forth
† Baseball, soccer, basketball, wrestling, and so forth.
‡ Cross country, track, tennis, crew, swimming, and so forth.
§ Bowling, golf, archery, field events, and so forth.
†† No exclusions.
‖ Each patient should be judged on an individual basis in conjunction with a cardiologist and surgeon.

Conditions	Colli-sion°	Contact†	Non-contact‡	Other§
Skin				
Boils, impetigo, and herpes simplex gladiatorum	X	X		
Spleen, enlarged	X	X		
Hernia				
Inguinal or femoral hernia	X	X	X	
Musculoskeletal				
Symptomatic abnormalities or inflammations	X	X	X	X
Functional inadequacy of the musculoskeletal system, congenital or acquired, incompatible with the contact or skill demands of the sport	X	X	X	
Neurologic				
History or symptoms of previous serious head trauma or repeated concussions	X			
Controlled convulsive disorder	¶	¶	¶	¶
Convulsive disorder not moderately well controlled by medication	X			
Previous surgery on head	X	X		
Renal				
Absence of one kidney	X	X		
Renal disease	X	X	X	X
Genitalia				
Absence of one testicle	° °	° °	° °	° °
Undescended testicle	° °	° °	° °	° °

¶ Each patient should be judged on an individual basis. All things being equal, it is probably better to encourage a young boy or girl to participate in a noncontact sport rather than a contact sport. However, if a patient has a desire to play a contact sport and this is deemed a major ameliorating factor in his or her adjustment to school, associates, and the seizure disorder, serious consideration should be given to letting him or her participate if the seizures are moderately well controlled or the patient is under good medical management.

°° The Committee approves the concept of contact sports participation for youths with only one testicle or with an undescended testicle(s), except in specific instances such as an inguinal canal undescended testicle(s), following appropriate medical evaluation to rule out unusual injury risk. However, the athlete, parents, and school authorities should be fully informed that participation in contact sports for youths with only one testicle carries a slight injury risk to the remaining healthy testicle. Fertility may be adversely affected following an injury. But the chances of an injury to a descended testicle are rare, and the injury risk can be further substantially minimized with an athletic supporter and protective device.

5
■■■■■

The Dangerous Side of Sports Play

When our children become involved in organized sports, we take on a responsibility for their well-being that begins in the home, extends to the sidelines, and continues even through the off-season. But sometimes, despite our best efforts, young athletes get caught up in the dangerous side of sports play that jeopardizes their health and undermines their efforts to achieve optimal performance levels. The problem areas young athletes commonly encounter include rapid weight loss, excessive weight gain, anorexia nervosa, bulimia, anabolic steroid use, and sports burnout. Knowing about these problems and being able to recognize their symptoms is an important aspect of injury and illness prevention.

Rapid Weight Loss

Rapid weight loss can be defined as a loss of more than two to three pounds a week. Athletes will commonly try to lose weight quickly to participate in weight-matched sports such as wrestling, boxing, and youth-league football. Runners, gymnasts, dancers, and figure skaters have also been known to knock off weight just before a competition in the misguided belief that lower body weight equals improved athletic performance.

Joe, for example, wanted to wrestle on the high school's varsity team. At 136 pounds, however, he was too heavy to win the only open spot, which was in the lightweight division. So with three days until the first weigh-in, Joe went on a "crash" diet to lose 10 pounds. Joe's teammates encouraged his efforts and gave him this popular weight-loss method:

1. Eat only fruit and one candy bar each day (rumor had it that fruit gave low-calorie nutrition and chocolate gave energy).
2. Put on a rubber suit, use an electric heater to heat the room to 110 degrees, and exercise excessively to sweat off the pounds.
3. Use laxatives to get rid of "extra" food held in the intestines and induce vomiting to empty the stomach.

After three days on this program, Joe weighed in at 119 pounds and 14 ounces. He had earned the coveted spot on the varsity team. Joe's next challenge will be to keep the weight off so he will make weight before every match, and at the same time stay healthy and strong enough to wrestle competitively. Unfortunately, this is not likely to happen. Rapid weight loss does not enhance health or give athletes the competitive edge; it makes them prone to injury and illness.

Dehydration Diets

Although body fat determines a person's weight, athletes in a hurry find it easier and faster to drop pounds by shedding water weight rather than body fat. They do this with dehydration diets like Joe's that restrict fluid intake and take water from the body through vomit, sweat, and spit. If these methods don't work fast enough, some will then use enemas and laxatives to further rid the body of fluids.

There are many reasons to condemn this kind of weight loss. As explained in Chapter Two, the body needs a full supply of water to function properly; it needs water to bring oxygen and nutrients to all parts of the body, to allow for elimination of body waste, to transport the heat generated by active muscles to the skin's surface, and to eliminate the heat from the body through sweat. Dehydration puts the athlete in a compromised state, and continued water loss causes many dangerous changes in the body's ability to function. It decreases the blood volume and plasma and reduces the heart output. It restricts the blood flow through the kidneys and diminishes muscular strength. It also makes the athlete prone to heat stroke or exhaustion, fever, nausea, general body weakness, and diminished physical performance.

Sports-related dehydration diets are especially dangerous if the athlete expects to keep the weight off. Because one glass of water will add on weight, the athlete will need to continue the water deprivation to maintain the lower weight. Each day without appropriate water intake further reduces the body's ability to function properly. Wrestlers and boxers often fall into this trap because they must weigh in before every match and because some believe they will have the advantage over smaller competitors in the lower weight class. Some get in the habit of practicing dehydration techniques one or two days before every match and then returning to normal eating and drinking patterns until two days before the next match. This fluctuation in body weight is upsetting to the athlete's body systems. Weight fluctuation is also dangerous for young athletes who attempt to compete in the same weight class year after year. Obviously, as their bodies grow and mature they put on additional weight. Trying to drop that weight when sports season rolls around plays havoc with the body's efforts to grow.

If your young athlete plays a weight-matched sport, watch for these signs of intentional dehydration:

- exercising in a rubber suit
- turning up the room temperature while exercising
- using the sauna to "relax"
- refusing to drink anything
- using diuretics or cathartics

Athletes who try to lose weight rapidly lose sight of the importance of going into competition with maximum levels of strength, endurance, and speed. They need to know the bottom line. You can not reduce rapidly without sacrificing normal growth and reducing muscle strength and function. The Reducing Diet Guidelines on page 98 will show your athlete how to lose weight safely.

Overweight Athletes

Children who are overweight should certainly lose weight because that is best for their overall health. Moreover, studies have shown that overweight athletes do not recover from injury as easily or quickly as do their lighter teammates. Extra pounds put additional stress on the joints and that makes rehabilitation more difficult. For example, every step you take puts three times the body's weight biomechanically through the knee joint. The joint of a 115-pound person can withstand the 345 pounds of force without stress; but if that same athlete were just 15 pounds overweight, it would add an additional 45 pounds of stress to the same joint. Obviously, the injured knee will not heal as easily or quickly as it should.

Overweight children should lose weight, but they should not shed pounds too quickly. Reduction diets should set a goal of gradual weight loss, and they need to be carefully supervised because growing bodies must have balanced and varied diets. The following general guidelines will help you establish a safe reducing diet and they will give you an indication of whether you need your doctor's help to monitor the progress.

REDUCING DIET GUIDELINES

1. Athletes should never lose more than two or three pounds per week.
2. Caloric intake must not go below 2,000 calories per day.
3. The reduced calories should not jeopardize a well-balanced diet and reduce the child's ability to perform at an optimal level in athletics, school, and recreational activities.
4. The diet should be closely supervised on a daily basis.
5. A reducing diet should be based on a negative balance of energy that allows for caloric restriction from reduced food intake and caloric consumption from increased exercise.
6. Weight goals should be set six to eight weeks in advance of the sport season.

Losing Extra Body Fat

You may be surprised when your seemingly "perfect weight" athletes announce that the coach wants them to lose weight. If this happens you will need to find out more about your athlete's body composition to determine if he or she can safely afford to lose some weight.

How can you tell if your "slim" child has excess body fat? The answer is a bit complex because height and weight tables (like those developed by insurance companies to weed out obese applicants) are generally inaccurate, very often invalid, and don't explain weight in terms of body composition. Body weight is comprised of lean mass (bone, muscle, and water which can not be reduced) and fat (which may be in greater supply then needed). Fat is necessary for healthy body functioning; it stores energy, insulates nerves, protects vital organs, and helps in normalizing one's metabolism. But most children have more than they need. Athletic boys, for example, usually have 8 to 12 percent body fat, but the ideal fat content for boys is 4 to 5 percent of their total body weight. Athletic girls, in general, are 16 to 22 percent fat, yet need only 10 to 12 percent fat. Too much fat makes it harder for a person to move around and it forces the heart to work harder to circulate blood. Excess fat can also put strain on the knee, ankle, and hip joints. So if seemingly lean athletes find that they have excess body fat, they can safely lose weight and yet maintain maximum strength, endurance, and quickness by following the Reducing Diet Guidelines on page 98.

Unfortunately, although determination of body fat percentage is an excellent indication of optimal weight for competing athletes, this information means nothing unless you have some means of measuring fat. If you need to find your child's "correct" body weight, you may have to scout around for a coach, trainer, or doctor who has the knowledge, experience, and skill to evaluate a person's body fat composition accurately. Your best bet is to call a sports clinic or sports-medicine center at the local college or hospital to find such an expert.

This type of evaluation is done in one of two ways. An underwater weighing test can be used to determine body fat levels. In this test the athlete is submerged under water and the body fat composition is determined by either weighing the water that is displaced by the person's body, or by directly weighing him or her under the water. A more effective, accurate, and easily produced method is called skinfold analysis. In this kind of evaluation, specially designed calipers lift folds of skin and underlying fat from various body sites. (Lange or Herpenden calipers are widely used and recommended.) The thickness of these skinfolds, measured in millimeters, is calculated into a formula to determine the percentage of fat in the tissue.

Body fat analysis has become a common component of pre-season conditioning programs for professional athletes and even for athletes in some exceptional high schools. But for most parents the decision to allow their young athletes to diet or not to diet must come down to common sense and good judgment. If you feel that your child's health and athletic performance might be improved by a reduction in body weight, then begin a carefully monitored program that follows the Reducing Diet Guidelines on page 98 and incorporates the daily nutritional needs explained in Chapter Two.

Excessive Weight Gain

Some athletes (especially thin boys) feel they'd be better competitors if they were bigger, so they decide to "bulk up" by eating excessive amounts of fattening foods. They make a daily ritual of stuffing their bodies with cakes and pies and candies. If your son or daughter has decided to practice gluttony in the name of athletic enhancement, he or she needs to learn more about the relationship between body composition and sports performance.

Getting fatter will not improve anyone's athletic abilities and it contradicts efforts to stay healthy. Body fat is nothing more than fat. The vast majority of American boys and girls have more body fat than they need for healthy body functioning. Adding more fat to the body compromises quickness and limits performance. It also jeopardizes good health by adding volume to existing fat cells and raising cholesterol levels; long after children have matured, filled out, and grown to their full size, they carry these excess fat cells and artery-clogging cholesterol deposits into adulthood.

If your athletes feel they are skinny and want to gain weight, help them do it in a safe way by following these guidelines:

SAFE WEIGHT GAIN SYSTEM

1. Maintain a well-balanced daily diet.
2. Increase caloric intake by no more than 1000 calories each day.
3. Increase intake of complex carbohydrates such as whole wheat breads, low-sugar cereals, pasta, rice, potatoes, carrots, fruits, and nuts.
4. Reduce intake of animal fats like meat, butter and eggs, and limit salty foods such as pretzels, popcorn, corn chips that hold extra water.

This kind of diet will give your children a few additional healthy pounds. But even after initial weight gain, you may find that what they really want is larger muscle mass. Unfortunately, as explained in Chapter Three, girls and prepubescent boys do not have the male hormone testosterone that's needed to increase muscle size. And even after puberty, body building for boys is a slow process that requires an ongoing training program. That's why athletes who are in a hurry to build muscles may be easily influenced by their friends to use dangerous body-building devices such as weight-on pills and formulas, over-training programs, and even anabolic steroids (see page 107 for a full discussion of these dangerous drugs). The diets and growth patterns of highly competitive athletes and of those obsessed with their personal body image should be watched closely. Warning signs of weight-gain abuse include:

- a sudden change of diet to include monstrous portions of "fattening" foods
- gulping pills called "vitamins" which may actually be weight-gain supplements or anabolic steroids
- growth of muscle mass in girls and prepubescent boys

- use of powdered supplements that do little to sustain weight gain
- development of more than one to two pounds of muscle mass per week in older high school boys engaged in weight training

If your young athletes insist that they need to gain weight, you can help them add on a few pounds by increasing their daily caloric intake of nutritious foods. But after that you'll need to help them accept that sometimes only the passage of time can make the body grow and mature.

Anorexia Nervosa

Some athletes lose weight in a conscientious effort to enhance their athletic performance, but they then develop such a terrifying fear of gaining weight that they continue to "diet" and shed body fat that their bodies need for survival. These athletes, who are most often female°, may develop sports-related anorexia nervosa.

Fifteen-year-old Heather was an attractive, intelligent, and popular track star. Her coaches knew she had that extra something that would earn her trophies, championships, and eventually a lucrative college scholarship. As she finished her freshman season, the varsity coach took Heather aside to compliment her talent and to assure her of a place on the varsity team the following year. He also asked her to follow a prescribed off-season conditioning program that would bring her to the field in top shape. As a parting comment the coach, half-jokingly, called over his shoulder, "And stay away from the sweet stuff, Heather. A track star needs to be lean."

Heather was thrilled by the coach's attention and she was determined to live up to his expectations. With the enthusiasm of an Olympic hopeful, she immediately threw herself into

° Because eating disorders primarily affect females we will use the pronoun "she" throughout this section.

the suggested program of exercises and put herself on a strict reducing diet. After two weeks, however, Heather still felt out of shape and fat. She doubled her daily exercise time and decided to eat nothing but two apples a day until she had a "lean" body. Several months later, weak and emaciated, Heather was hospitalized and fed against her will intravenously. Once in top shape and perfect health, Heather was now unable to walk even a few feet without suffering total exhaustion; she was suffering from anorexia nervosa.

Anorexia nervosa is an eating disorder characterized by self-imposed starvation. Studies have consistently found that individuals most prone to this illness are females between the ages of 12 and 25 who come from middle- and upper-class homes, and who are bright, artistic, and self-disciplined. Although certainly not limited to any one sport, this eating disorder is more likely to affect athletes like gymnasts, dancers (especially ballerinas), and runners, whose performances are compromised by excess fat.

The exact causes of anorexia are unknown, but it is believed to be based on a psychological need for perfection and self-control. Anorexic girls are generally anxious to please and want to be the best in their sport, among their friends, and in their parents' eyes. As in Heather's case, sometimes it takes only an offhand remark, or an overheard comment about excess weight, or a mere suggestion to trigger the onset of self-imposed starvation. Families and coaches should know that pressing a young girl to strive for perfection in performance or body size contributes to the anorexic's struggle. The role that families and coaches play in fostering this disease is well illustrated in dancer Gelsey Kirkland's book, *Dancing on My Grave* (Doubleday). It is also being publicized by Olympic gymnast Cathy Rigby, who now speaks openly about her own battle with eating disorders.

The signs and symptoms of anorexia nervosa include 1) abnormal social isolation and withdrawal from family and friends; 2) lack of confidence in abilities; 3) ritualistic eating behavior, such as organizing food on a plate or dawdling over food; 4) obsession with counting calories; 5) excessive exercise in an effort to expend calories, often right before a meal; 6) related disorders, such as malnutrition, significant weight loss, dry skin, brittle hair, amenorrhea (interruption of normal menstrual cycle), or general malaise; 7) obsession with weighing oneself; and 8) overestimation of body size (seeing oneself as wider and fatter than one really is).[1]

Detection of these symptoms of anorexia is a cause for concern. Untreated, this disease can cause severe physical impairment, even death. The starved body needs immediate medical attention, and the athlete also needs prompt psychological counseling to deal with the underlying emotional problems. The sooner counseling begins, the better the chance of complete recovery.

Bulimia

Bulimia is an eating disorder characterized by a binge-purge syndrome. Bulimics binge on inordinate amounts of food (even when they're not hungry); then, feeling guilty for having eaten so much and fearful of weight gain, they purge their bodies through self-induced vomiting or with excessive use of diuretics and laxatives. The frequency of this binge-purge cycle varies from individual to individual. Some binge and purge only on weekends or only in response to stress; others binge-purge several times a day. But usually once the cycle is begun it rapidly increases in frequency. The amount of food ingested during a binge will also increase as the cravings grow stronger and last longer. It would not be unusual for a bulimic to eat two dozen cupcakes, two quarts of ice cream, and a very large meal at one sitting.

Like anorexics, bulimics tend to exercise obsessively. They see exercise as another form of purging calories from their bodies. This exercise addiction may appear at first to be an admirable trait in a young athlete. Body conditioning, after all, prevents injury and illness. But the obsessive exerciser uses exercise as a means of gaining permission to eat. "I'll eat this piece of bread," she may say to herself, "but then I'll run an extra five laps at today's practice." If something should happen to keep this athlete from running those extra five laps she will feel intense anxiety, self-loathing, and depression. This athlete has developed a variation of bulimia which psychologists have dubbed exercise bulimia.

Also like anorexics, bulimics are most often young perfection-seeking females who have some common psychological traits. The Association for Bulimia and Related Disorders in New York City describes the typical bulimia victim as follows:

> Bulimics are usually well-groomed, attractive, outgoing young ladies who do not appear to have a significant weight problem. Thousands of American women between adolescence and mid-adulthood have this disorder. Most bulimics are overly concerned with a perfect presentation of themselves.
>
> They suffer from low-self-esteem and disproportionate need for validation from important others. This perfect facade masks underlying needs and emotional discomfort. They are sensitive to rejection and are often bewildered when their perfect presentation does not result in the acceptance they are looking for. They turn to food as a means of nurturing themselves, perhaps turning from the outer world in anger or disappointment.
>
> The binging is initially a pleasurable release from the unusual control and constant self-monitoring. However, the overeating is immediately followed by guilt, shame, and remorse; thus the purging. The purge begins a renewed drive for perfection and initiates yet another false attempt at controlling one's world.
>
> Bulimics are not only unassertive victims in their relationships with others (whom they continually try to please) but are also victims of the binge-purge cycle, which for many totally controls their lives.[2]

Unlike girls with anorexia, bulimics are not found exclusively among the middle and upper classes. Bulimia knows no class or income barrier. All young female athletes who want to achieve success, please their parents and coaches, and who possess the psychological characteristics stated above are capable of becoming bulimics. Also unlike anorexics, girls with bulimia may not stand out because of a skeleton-like appearance. They generally maintain a normal body weight, and their families may marvel that they can eat so much and not gain weight. Most of the binging is done in private, and the purging is a sacred secret; and the physical changes are more subtle than those associated with anorexia.

SIGNS AND SYMPTOMS OF BULIMIA

1. A persistent sore throat from constant vomiting.
2. A round, puffy, and bloated face as a result of recurrent regurgitation, which may cause the salivary glands to become infected and swollen.
3. Dehydration and dry skin.
4. Constipation because the body doesn't have sufficient fluid after purging.
5. Muscle spasms, kidney problems, or cardiac arrest, which can be brought on by an electrolyte imbalance caused by loss of body fluids.
6. Abdominal bloating.
7. Tooth decay caused by inadequate nutrition, frequent vomiting, and a lack of protein in the diet.

Bulimia and anorexia are dangerous eating disorders that can certainly keep young athletes from reaching their full potential and make them prone to injury and illness. Some victims carry the disorder into adulthood; others die. But still others, with appropriate medical and psychological treatment, are cured. If you want more information about these eating disorders contact your doctor and one of these organizations:

- National Association of Anorexia Nervosa and Associated Disorders, P.O. Box 7, Highland Park, Illinois 60035; telephone 312-831-3438.
- Anorexia Nervosa and Related Eating Disorders, Inc., P.O. Box 5102, Eugene, Oregon 97405; telephone 503-344-1144.
- American Anorexia/Bulimia Association, Inc., 133 Cedar Lane, Teaneck, New Jersey 07666.

Anabolic Steroid Use

Seventeen-year-old Rich is a powerful linebacker on the varsity football team. He has exceptional speed and muscular strength and size. Rich and his coaches feel that his success is due to three years of intensive weight training. Rich's parents are also proud of his athletic accomplishments but they are worried. They've noticed that although Rich's weight-lifting has certainly increased his muscle size, he hasn't grown in height in the last two years. They have also watched his mild-mannered personality change into a short-tempered volatile one. His mom is also upset that Rich has decided to grow a beard to cover up his acne. "He seems too young to have such thick facial hair," she has told their family doctor, "and I don't understand why he refuses to go to a dermatologist for acne treatment." Rich's parents seem to be grappling with problems typical in raising a teenager. But in this case the problems are not typical. Rich's large muscles, stunted growth, change in personality, heavy facial hair, and acne are all caused by his abuse of anabolic steroids.

Steroids are not in themselves bad or dangerous. They are a group of powerful synthetic substances that resemble the male sex hormone, testosterone, which is produced naturally by the male's testes. Synthetic steroids were first developed in the 1930s in an attempt to build body tissue and prevent the breakdown of tissue that occurs in some debilitating diseases. Although the Federal Drug Administration has since found that anabolic steroids do not effectively reach these goals, the drugs are approved and legally prescribed for treatment of certain types of anemia, certain kinds of breast cancer in women, and hereditary angioedema (a type of allergic reaction to some insect bites and foods).

Steroids become injurious to health and even deadly when they are used nonmedically and illegally to enhance body size and athletic performance. It is believed that these drugs were first used in athletics by the Russians in 1954, when Soviet athletes dominated many international sports events. To remain competitive, in the late 1950s many American athletes followed suit. Today steroids are widely abused by professional, amateur, high school, and even junior high school male and female athletes who seek bigger muscles and superior physical performance.

The exact number of athletes who abuse steroids is unknown because nonmedical use is illegal and therefore no one publicizes its use. But as college, professional, and Olympic teams begin to require steroid testing before competitions, the large number of athletes involved in steroid use is beginning to come to light. In the most celebrated case in recent years, track star Ben Johnson was stripped of his 1989 Olympic gold medal in the 100-yard dash when his steroid test came back positive. On the football field, Brian Bosworth, a University of Oklahoma All-American, was barred from the 1986 bowl game because he also tested positive. Then in 1987 the National Football League, recognizing the problem, set down rules that call for steroid testing in training camps and require players who test positive to be sidelined for 30 days and to be barred from the league after two additional positive readings.

As steroid use by athletic role models and sports idols continues to make headlines, it becomes easy to see that the use of these drugs is no longer confined to dingy smelly gyms where obsessive body builders secretively load up in dark corners. Steroid abuse has crept into all American sports and is openly practiced in posh health spas, fitness centers, local gymnasiums, and even high school locker rooms. In fact, a 1988 survey found that 6.6 percent of male high school seniors have used steroids, and that 40 percent of these boys began using the drugs before they reached the age of sixteen.[3]

Why would talented young athletes, many of whom would never think of abusing alcohol, crack, cocaine, or marijuana, take steroids? A piece of the complex answer lies in the nature of sports competition. Athletics place great emphasis on body composition, weight, and appearance. In overly competitive environments athletes are sometimes tempted to alter their physical make-up and size to improve their performance, impress their peers, please their coaches and parents, and make them better than their opponents (or merely equal if they believe their opponents are taking the drugs). They see others taking the drugs in pill form or by injection and they see only the positive effects: a sense of euphoria, an aggressive and vigorous attitude, larger muscle size in less training time, and increased amounts of energy and speed.

What they don't immediately see are the negative body changes that steroid abuse can cause. One such body change actually *causes* sports-related injuries. It has been found that users have an increased chance of injury to muscles, tendons, and ligaments. Although steroids give mass to the muscles, they do not strengthen the muscle supports. When muscles get too heavy for their supports they are prone to injury and then do not heal as well or as quickly as they do if they have developed naturally.

Also, "roids," "juice," or "gas," as steroids are called, cause dangerous side effects in one-third to one-half of the people who use them. (These numbers may be higher, but the long-term effects on users who take the drugs over a long period of time are still unknown.) Steroid use stimulates the hypothalamus area of the brain, which in turn affects other areas of the brain and body—most particularly the pituitary gland, the male testes, and the female reproductive organs. In males, this can cause decreased sperm production and a reduction in the size of the testes. This can lead to testicular cancer, infertility and/or sterility. Male athletes may also notice female-like breast tissue development. These side effects may be transient during the period of steroid use or they may become permanent conditions. Female athletes who abuse steroids may notice the development of male-patterned baldness, facial hair growth, deepening of the voice, and a decrease in breast size. Unfortunately for the female, most steroid abuse side effects are irreversible.

After an athlete reaches skeletal maturity, steroid use can cause a side effect that mimics the symptoms of a pituitary gland tumor. This condition, known as acromegaly, increases the width of bone and connective tissues, which causes grotesque feature changes on the body and face. This condition is responsible for the physical appearance of personalities such as Lurch on the TV show "The Adams Family," and the wrestler Andre the Giant.

Steroid abuse has other far-reaching effects that athletes may not appreciate at an early age. These synthetic hormones can adversely affect the body's production of high-density lipo proteins (HDL), a form of cholesterol that decreases the risk factors of the dangerous low-density lipo (LDL) proteins. Without full production of proteins HDL, the athlete is at increased risk for heart attack in later life. Steroids also endanger the long-term health of athletes who are already in a compromised state because they are anemic or have sickle cell anemia. Steroids use will aggravate these pre-existing problems and may eventually cause fatal liver or kidney disease.

Chart 5.1 lists these and other physical side effects that are attributable to steroid use. In addition to bodily changes, users may also suffer psychological problems such as mood depression, nervous tension, irritability, hostility, aggression, sleep problems, delusions, and even suicidal tendencies. Obviously, steroids are not the wonder drug they may at first seem to be to your young athlete.

To many young athletes the positive side of steroid use looks too good to pass up. That's why parents and coaches need to educate them about the bad side. Tell them what their friends won't—that as soon as the user stops taking the drugs, the extra weight and muscle mass are quickly lost, but

CHART 5.1
SOME PHYSICAL SIDE-EFFECTS OF ANABOLIC STEROID ABUSE

acne (Unaware of the cause, a dermatologist may prescribe medications such as tetracycline or isotretinoin which will aggravate the existing side-effects.)
breast development in males
cancer of the liver
cholesterol increase
clitoris enlargement in females
death
decreased sperm count (reversible)
decrease in women's breast size (irreversible)
dizziness
edema (water retention)
frequent or continuing and sometimes painful penile erection
headaches
heart disease
hairiness in women (irreversible)
increased blood pressure
jaundice (yellowing of the skin and whites of the eyes)
kidney disease
liver disease and tumors
male-pattern baldness in women (irreversible)
menstrual irregularities
muscle cramps
nausea and vomiting
oily skin and hair
premature epiphyseal closure in young people (This will stunt growth and the user will never achieve full growth potential.)
prostate enlargement
sterility (reversible)
swelling of feet or lower legs
testicular atrophy

many of the negative effects stay behind. Inform them that steroids are physically and psychologically addictive, and tell them that the college teams don't want them if their athletic performance is the result of "juice" rather than natural ability. Assure them that you want them to be involved in sports, that you support and encourage their efforts, but insist that steroid use not be a part of their training. Openly discuss the ethical issues of steroid use: focus on cheating—cheating in the sport, cheating fellow athletes, and cheating one's own body. Let there be no doubt that because you love them, you will jump in to play interference the moment you feel anything but hard work and effort is behind muscle growth and physical performance.

If you are worried that your child is abusing steroids, discuss your suspicions with your family physician. Then arrange an opportunity for your athlete to discuss steroid use with the doctor. The physician can objectively point out negative side effects, can administer a blood test to detect steroid use, and can determine if any steroid-related conditions, such as hypertension or abnormal liver or kidney function, are already present.

Sports Burnout

Sports participation is good for kids; it increases their concept of self-worth and promotes lifelong fitness habits. Right? Well, sometimes, unfortunately, No: sports participation can put a great deal of stress on a young athlete and cause psychological harm and physical injury. Throughout this century psychologists have studied the benefits and risks of participation in organized sports programs. They have warned parents, coaches, and physical education teachers about the negative effects of overzealous competitions, of overly strenuous training, and of pressure to reach high expectations. All of these things, say the psychologists, lead to what we now call sports burnout.

Kids drop out of sports for a variety of reasons. Some factors associated with age and development are the following:

- Many kids quit sports at ages 6 to 8 because these children are interested in the process—not the result—of things.[4] They enjoy swinging the bat, throwing the football, and kicking the soccer ball. The trying and the doing are fun. But when parents and coaches step in and show anger and disappointment because the action didn't lead to the expected result of a base hit, gained yardage, or a goal, kids may decide that sports play is not fun after all.
- At ages 9 and 10, young people are just beginning to understand the importance of teamwork, desire, and concentration. If this awareness is fostered and developed, children can grow to be cooperative and determined athletes. But parents and coaches who can't tolerate age-appropriate mind-wandering and the me-first mania that occasionally mixes with an "I'm too tired and I don't want to do this today" attitude, put undue pressure on these young athletes to behave and perform as little adults. This pushes them out of sports.
- From ages 11 through 13, kids start to make physical and social comparisons. This is a time of particularly high drop-out rates in sports, especially among girls. Kids who, given a few more years of physical growth and skill practice, might grow to be excellent athletes, drop out because they decide they're not good enough.[5]

Burnout is not caused by sports participation. It is caused by the competitive environment and the win-at-all-costs attitude forced on young athletes by adults. That's why, to foster a healthy atmosphere of sports play, you were asked in Chapter One to take a close look at your own attitude toward your child's sports participation. You were also advised to evaluate the coach's view of playing and winning. If parents and coaches both put enjoyment of the sport, the learning of skills, teamwork with friends, and good sportsmanship above winning, many more young athletes would stay in sports programs and would still be active ten, twenty, even thirty years down the line.

Some athletes are more prone to burnout than others. Highly susceptible athletes are often accomplished performers who set high, sometimes unrealistic, goals for themselves. They tend to invest a great deal of time and effort trying to meet these goals. They usually don't react well to criticism; they may have a weak support system and will often suffer from boredom if the training regime is too repetitious.

Signs of sports burnout include:

- pleas of helplessness if the athlete doesn't achieve the goals he or she sets
- a lack of self-esteem
- increased physical frailness
- anxiety
- depression
- fatigue
- insomnia
- withdrawal
- declining athletic performance

These clinical signs indicate possible sports burnout, but if your young athlete suffers these symptoms he or she should have a medical check-up before you conclude they are caused solely by stress. These symptoms are similar to those of a variety of diseases, including neuromusculoskeletal problems, undiagnosed heart or lung problems, kidney ailments, and anemia. You must have a physician rule out these problems before you can appropriately and effectively address the problem of burnout.

Sports burnout causes many young athletes to lose interest in sports, and others to lose their positive self-image. When fun is ignored in favor of intense workouts, sports burnout can also be responsible for causing sports-related physical injuries due to overtraining. The signs of overtraining are detailed on page 65 and include fatigue, decrease in motivation, and chronic soreness. This soreness can be a symptom of an overuse injury (page 221). Physicians are noting a rise in such injuries and suspect that they are caused by the strenuous, repetitious training activities that seem to be in vogue among championship-bound youth sport leagues.

Physicians have also noticed a growing trend in burned-out athletes who try to hold onto the pain of an injury. Sixteen-year-old Julie was admitted four times in one month to Boston's Children's Hospital for severe right foot pain.[6] Julie had been an avid athlete who participated in her school's gymnastics and track programs. One year before her recent hospital admissions Julie had hurt her foot in gym class. The injury was described as a relatively minor sprain that healed well with Ace bandaging and weight-bearing restrictions. When Julie continued to complain of pain, her doctor prescribed a variety of therapeutic measures including exercises and whirlpool massage. The pain continued, so Julie's doctor suggested a psychological assessment to determine if emotional problems might be contributing to her pain. It was found that Julie's injury had occurred at the same time she had begun to lose athletic contests. She eventually admitted that her injury gave her medical protection from pressure to fulfill the expectations of friends and rejoin her sports teams. Julie was suffering real pain caused by a psychological pain syndrome. The number of such cases is rising each year and, regrettably, a disproportionately high number of these children sustain the initial injury in sports competition or training.

A psychological pain syndrome is suspect when, despite appropriate treatment, relatively minor injuries such as sprained ankles or tendonitis of the ankle, knee, or shoulder do not "heal." The young athlete will continue to complain of severe discomfort and will be unable to return to sports play even when medically cleared to do so. Not surprisingly, when these athletes can no longer hide behind the injury and must return to sports participation, they are very likely to suffer another injury. These stressed athletes may become accident-prone and after a history of minor injuries may progress to overt self-destruction and sustain a major debilitating injury.

Pressure to excel and to win affects young athletes in different ways. Some face the stress by trying harder and becoming more adept. Others push themselves beyond their capabilities and suffer overuse injuries. Some just plain quit, and a growing number of others find a socially acceptable way to "save face" and escape from the strain of competition by becoming and then staying injured.

Stress Management

The dangerous side of sports play generally encroaches on an athlete's enjoyment of physical activity when the fun of the game is lost in the struggle to win. You can enhance all that is positive about youth athletics by teaching your child how to deal with the stress of competition. The following relaxation exercises can be practiced before and during training periods and competitive events. They enable the athlete's body to better cope with the natural physical drain caused by stress and focus instead on their performance.

Deep Breathing Exercise

Because the body needs oxygen to fuel its stress response, athletes may take many short, quick breaths when they get tense. Some may even hyperventilate. Teach your young athlete how to short-circuit this stress response by regaining control of his or her breathing with the following deep breathing exercise.

- To stop the rapid breathing accompanying a stress response, first put your hand on your stomach.
- Then take a deep breath from the bottom of your stomach.

You should be able to feel your hand rise with your stomach muscles.

- Breathe in as you silently count to five.
- Let the air go out gently as you again count to five.
- Do this sequence two times in a row.
- Then breathe in a regular rhythmic and comfortable pattern.
- After a minute or two, follow the deep breathing sequence again.
- Repeat this deep-breathing/regular-breathing cycle two or three times (or as often as needed) until you find your breathing has returned to a natural and comfortable pace.

This deep breathing exercise can be practiced anywhere without anyone knowing that your athlete is engaged in a stress reduction technique. It is a quick and easy way to change the body's reaction to stress.

Progressive Muscle Relaxation

Athletes who experience stress through headaches, stomach cramps, stiff neck muscles, and so forth can use progressive muscle relaxation to calm the stress response that gets them "tied up in knots." To relax tense muscles effectively when anxiety strikes, your athlete should practice this muscle relaxation exercise in advance. Then when the muscles begin to tense during sports play, he or she will be able to identify the location of the tension and stop the stress attack.

To begin, tense and relax the various muscle groups listed below. Maintain that tension for fifteen seconds so you have time to feel how whole parts of your body are involved in tension. When you have a muscle group tensed, let your mind's eye experience that part of your body. If you're tensing your arm, for example, press your forearm down against the table. Feel when the tension goes out through your fingertips, up onto your shoulders, right into your neck—then relax.

Feel the experience of letting go—of consciously relaxing your muscles.

RELAXATION EXERCISE

Repeat this exercise three times each day with these muscle groups:

1. right hand	make a fist
right forearm	press down
2. left hand	make a fist
left forearm	press down
3. shoulders	shrug
4. neck	lean your head back and roll it from side to side
5. head:	
jaw	bite down lightly
tongue	press on the roof of your mouth
eyes	squint
forehead	frown and raise your brows
6. abdomen	tighten your stomach as if someone were going to hit you
7. back	press down on the floor
8. right leg	press down on the floor
left leg	press down on the floor
9. toes	curl under

Thought Control

Athletes can generate stress simply by thinking negative thoughts. If your sons or daughters allow themselves to dwell on their inadequacies or failures, they will undoubtedly open themselves up to stress-related sports injuries. The athletes who say to themselves, "I can't do this," "Everyone will make fun of me," "I know I'm going to lose the game for the team," "I'm a terrible player; I shouldn't even be here," are the ones most open to the dangerous side of sports play. Teach your athletes to think positive thoughts. If they find themselves looking on the gloomy side, encourage them to stop the thought immediately and replace it with a positive one. If, for example, you know your child is prone to worry, "I hope the coach doesn't watch me because I know I'll make a mistake," tell him or her to turn the thought around and think, "I hope the coach watches me because I know I'm good." The basis of thought control as a method of stress management is simple: when you talk to yourself, say something positive.

How ironic that sports play, which exists solely to enhance personal growth and development, can be a primary source of stress and unhappiness in young athletes. Keep in mind as your child progresses through organized sports programs that while some athletes cope well with the stress of competition and use it to raise their sense of self-esteem, others are not good losers and this puts them at risk for serious physical and psychological ailments. These athletes need your help, support, and guidance to get the most out of sports.

Part II
A Close Look at Specific Sports

6

■ ■ ■ ■ ■

Baseball/Softball

The origins of baseball go back into ancient history. There is evidence that the Egyptians of 5,000 years ago enjoyed batting contests with a club and ball. The British brought an early version of the game to this country in the early 1880s. American legend then gives credit to Abner Doubleday for having laid out the first U.S. baseball playing field at Cooperstown in New York in 1839.

One hundred years later, in 1939, the first official Little League game was played. Today Little League and other youth and high school baseball leagues comprise the largest youth sport in the world; several million boys and girls ages 6 to 18 play the game in over 25 countries.

Although baseball is a relatively safe sport, almost two percent of young baseball players are injured playing the game each year. The information in this chapter will help you keep your young baseball player healthy this season.

The mechanics of baseball safety are the same as those in softball. Although this chapter addresses the baseball player directly, the facts are equally applicable to softball players. There is a brief softball-specific discussion at the end.

123

Equipment

Batting Helmets

Batting helmets must have a NOCSAE (National Operating Committee on Standards for Athletic Equipment) seal on them to certify that they have been tested and judged to be safe. Quality helmets are padded and have flaps over *both* ears. Some players use helmets with polycarbonate face guards which protect the batter's face and yet do not interfere with vision. Any team member, other than a coach, who covers first or third base must also wear a protective helmet.

Catcher's Protective Gear

Catchers must wear protective equipment. They are required to wear 1) a chest protector (better-quality ones have a neck collar that guards the throat), 2) a catcher's mask with an attached throat protector, 3) a helmet that protects both the face and the back of the head from a swinging bat (some teams use a combination mask and helmet), and 4) shin guards (recommended ones protect the ankle, front and sides of the leg, and above the knee cap). These pieces of equipment should be worn at all times during practices and games when the athlete is actively playing the position. Also, any catcher warming up a pitcher on the sidelines or in between innings must wear a catcher's helmet and face mask.

Shoes

Youth-league players should wear flexible rubber-cleated shoes for safety reasons. Because these athletes are inexperienced in the skill of sliding, they are often cut by metal spikes. These cuts easily become infected because the spikes are dirty and harbor tetanus bacteria as well as the bacteria of the manure used to fertilize the grassy areas of the playing field.

Older players will probably wear metal spikes because they give better traction, but these players need to learn proper sliding and tagging techniques to avoid being injured by these kinds of shoes.

Athletic Supporter With Protective Cup

This piece of protective equipment is mandatory for boys who are catchers. It is optional, but recommended, for all other male players.

Bases

For preadolescent players, magnetized "break-away" bases are safer than ones anchored into the ground. These players often get hurt sliding improperly into immovable bases.

Baseballs

Find out if the league rules allow the use of softer balls for players age 12 and under. If so, petition to have your child's league switch to balls such as Worth Sports Company's R.I.F. (Reduced Injury Factor) ball. These can be ordered from Worth Inc., PO Box 550, Tullahoma, TN 37388, 615-455-0691. If these balls are not allowed, find out how the rule barring them can be changed. They can substantially reduce the risk of injury in youth-league baseball.

Sun Protection

Infielders and outfielders should use sunglasses or put black sun glare reflector under their eyes when necessary. This will help them see the ball and will prevent acute collision injuries. Because baseball is played outdoors in unshaded areas, fair-skinned players should wear a sun screen lotion to protect them from the sun's ultraviolet rays.

Practice

All practices should begin with a warm-up period. Young players need to develop the warm-up habit; adolescent players going through growth spurts need to enhance their flexibility to reduce the risk of injury; and older players need to warm up their muscles so their arms and shoulders can withstand the stress of forcible throwing and their legs endure the sudden sprinting required in base running.

Baseball is a very popular sport and so most teams have a number of players who "sit the bench." When you watch a practice session, make sure that all players are involved. Youth-league baseball loses an untold number of young athletes each year to boredom and sports burnout. This situation can be quickly remedied if all players have a chance to play and if the players rotate positions so that no one is continually stranded in the outfield. Numerous surveys attest that when young players have a choice between sitting the bench on a winning team or playing on a losing team, the vast majority choose the losing team. Sitting the bench is also physically dangerous for a player who, without proper training or conditioning, is suddenly called in to substitute for a starting player. To keep your athletes interested in sports and to reduce their risk of injury, shop around for a team and a coach that will give your young player plenty of action.

Mimicking professional teams, most baseball coaches create hand-signal communication systems. Find out what signals your child's team uses and help him or her practice. Players who don't understand or can't remember the signals are at risk for collision injuries.

Watch for enforcement of sideline protection rules. All players not on the field should be kept behind a protective screen. Batters in the "on-deck circle" should also be behind a protective screen. (Youth leagues should not allow batters to stand "on deck.")

Knowing and using proper technique is an important factor in injury prevention. Make sure that a part of each practice session is devoted to skill instruction. Because it is not uncommon for athletes in youth leagues to play a variety of positions each game, all players should learn the skills of all positions. The following are a sampling of the basic skills that should be taught to baseball players:

For Pitchers

Pitchers need to learn and practice each stage of the throw from the wind-up to recovery. Pitchers (especially those in the younger youth leagues) need to learn how to execute a proper overhand throw. Sidearm throwing should be discouraged because it puts increased stress across immature and growing bones which leads to "Little League elbow" (page 262). Curve balls in youth leagues are also the cause of arm injury. Pitching instruction should also emphasize the role of the legs in the throwing motion; proper use of the legs eases the strain on the throwing arm. All pitchers need to learn how to follow through after their pitch so they can recover quickly and protect themselves against the returning batted ball. Studies have found that upper extremity problems common to pitchers are often caused by improper deceleration (the motion used after the ball has been released).

For Fielders

Outfielders may stand on the field for extended periods of time without seeing any action. That's why they should repeat their warm-up routine between innings, and in cold weather they should be encouraged to move around in between pitches. This will keep their muscles warm and ready for action when they are suddenly called on to run after a ball and make a long throw. As explained in Chapter Three, cold muscles are most susceptible to injury.

All fielders should be taught specific safety skills. They should know how to call for a ball and how to shade their eyes from sun glare. They should also know how to tag runners without risking injury from being spiked or being run over. (All players, fielders and runners should avoid collisions at the plate.)

For Catchers

By the nature of their position, catchers are at increased risk for injury. Therefore they need special instruction in skill and safety techniques. First, catchers must have complete and proper-fitting equipment, as listed above. Then they must learn how to block pitches that hit the dirt and how to protect their hands from injury. Catchers should be discouraged from using their bodies to protect the plate against an opponent who is trying to score.

For Batters

All batters must wear a safety batting helmet every time they're up at bat. They may also want to wear batting gloves to protect their fingers. Players should spend time practicing how to get out of the way of a wild pitch so they don't get hit by the ball. They also need to learn the proper placement of the hands and fingers when attempting to bunt a ball. They then must practice how to discard the bat without throwing it after the ball is hit.

For Base Runners

Before getting up at bat, players should be encouraged to warm up and to take practice swings with the bat. They should also stretch the hamstrings and Achilles tendons (see conditioning recommendations below). Base runners must be taught how to slide properly to prevent leg or hand injuries. Because sliding (especially head-first sliding) can be dangerous, many youth leagues have rules against it.

Injuries

The majority of baseball-related injuries are caused by sudden trauma. Contusions (page 274) and abrasions (page 273) will sometimes happen when a player is hit by a ball or is bruised sliding into a base or diving to catch a ball. Fractures (page 235-237) and sprains (page 259) of the finger, leg, ankle, or wrist are most often caused by collision during base running. Finger dislocations (page 234) are often caused by improper catching.

Stress and overuse injuries are relatively rare in the sport of baseball. Occasionally, however, shin splints (page 239) may develop if players begin intensive practice without first preparing the leg muscles with adequate conditioning and warm-up (page 44). A common example of overuse syndrome can be found in "Little League elbow" (page 262); repetitive throwing at an early age and improper throwing technique can strain the muscle unit in the elbow.

See page 92 for a list of medical conditions that may prohibit participation in baseball.

Conditioning

Baseball is a game of skill that requires sharp eye-hand co-ordination and quick reflexes. Baseball players can improve their performance and protect themselves from injury by conditioning for:

flexibility (page 67): shoulders, arms, hamstrings, Achilles tendons, hips, lower back.
agility (page 71)
speed (page 71)
cardiovascular endurance (page 72)
strength (page 72): abdomen, legs, shoulders, wrist.

Baseball is a sport with a relatively low injury rate. Most injuries that do occur are preventable. Injuries such as overuse syndromes and throwing injuries are due to improper technique when hitting and running. These and avoidable collision injuries should be your targets of focus to ensure your young athlete's baseball season is an enjoyable and healthy one.

Softball

Softball is so similar to baseball in injury-related information that a separate chapter would be redundant. The discussion of baseball equipment, practices, injuries, and body conditioning presented above is equally applicable to the prevention of softball injuries, with these two exceptions. First, although "softer" softballs are not marketed for younger players, pre-adolescents can reduce their risk of injury and better learn the skills of throwing and catching if they are allowed to use the smaller, 10-inch ball. Second, because the underarm pitching motion does not strain the arm the way the overhand baseball throw does, softball pitchers are not limited in the number of consecutive innings or games they can pitch. With correct technique and proper warm-up of the shoulder and wrist, softball pitchers will not suffer the stress injuries found in baseball pitchers.

7

■ ■ ■ ■ ■

Basketball

Basketball, a sport popular among boys and girls alike, relies on learned skills of dribbling, shooting, passing, and rebounding. It demands tremendous physical ability to accelerate and change direction rapidly, to run at top speed for extended periods of time, to jump and throw, and to compete for possession of the ball. It is also a game that asks athletes to develop highly specialized individual skills and then use them cooperatively with teammates working toward the same goal. The information in this chapter outlines the aspects of sports participation that enable young players to do these things in a safe and enjoyable way.

Equipment

Ball

The basketball itself is obviously an important piece of equipment in this sport. The kind of ball used affects the player's ability to play the game safely and productively. Smaller sized balls are used in girls' leagues. The smaller size compensates for the relative lack of arm strength and it enables girls to maintain better control of the ball.

Girls' basketballs as well as standard balls vary in quality of composition and in buoyancy. Some balls, made for outdoor courts, are tougher and have a pitted surface. Others are made of leather for indoor courts and are smoother; they are more easily beat up if used on outdoor surfaces. The basketball that your young athlete uses should be one manufactured for the surface he or she plays on and it should not be old and worn. Once the ball is worn down to a smooth, slippery touch, the players can not properly grip, catch, dribble, pass, or shoot it. The ball should also be inflated properly so that the athletes are not straining to make a "dead" ball bounce or losing control of an over-inflated wild ball.

Shoes

The leather high-top basketball shoes that most players wear today are generally appropriate footwear for this game. The high-top gives the ankles additional support when they are laced properly, but make sure your young athlete knows that these shoes can increase the risk of ankle injury when they are very loosely laced or left untied as is sometimes the fashion today. Whether the athlete wears canvas or leather, high-top or low cut, it is most important that the shoe fits properly and has a sturdy sole and a well-cushioned arch.

Bra

A female player should wear a high-quality supportive bra. This will protect her breasts from painful contusions that can occur if she is elbowed in the chest by an opponent.

Athletic Supporter

A male player should wear an athletic supporter with a cup. This will protect his genital area from painful collision with an opponent's knee or elbow.

Knee Pads

Knee pads are worn as a matter of personal preference. Some players feel they give the knees more support but most wear them to protect the knees from floor burns and abrasions (page 273). Athletes who regularly fall down during their playing time on the court should ask the coach for a pair of knee pads. If the team can't supply them, you can buy your own at most sporting goods stores.

Practice

Basketball is a contact sport that is played, for the most part, without protective equipment. Therefore the players must rely on physical conditioning and skill to keep themselves from injury. To do this, practice sessions should emphasize body conditioning as well as learning and practicing the fundamentals, and then executing them with proper technique.

When you observe a basketball practice, check to be sure the players are in a safe environment. The court should be clean, because dusty or dirty floors promote slipping and falling. The court should also be clear of debris or other athletic equipment and apparatus. Players risk tripping and collision if the court is cluttered.

Because basketball makes exceptional physical demands on the body, all practices and games must begin with warm-ups. Encourage your young athletes to stretch out with the flexibility exercises listed below and to begin practice sessions with reduced speed and intensity. All players should be allowed to warm up their muscles gradually before giving 100 percent.

In the game of basketball only 5 players from each team are on the court at one time. Yet most teams have 10 to 15 players on the roster. Make sure that all players on your child's team are actively involved in the practice sessions. This will keep second-string players interested in the sport and it will keep them prepared and conditioned in the event that they are sent into a game.

Basketball is a game of sharp cuts and angles, of quick starts and stops, and of maximum control with minimum wasted motion. Therefore practices must emphasize footwork so players will not be injured when they make these moves on unconditioned muscle units. In addition to practicing footwork drills that simulate playing situations, make sure your young player knows how to keep his or her knees flexed with the feet spread comfortably apart and with the weight evenly distributed on the balls of the feet. No one can safely (or effectively) play basketball when the knees are locked or when bending at the waist.

Shooting skills are the most fun to practice, but these drills should do more than give kids a chance to throw balls at the hoop. Proper shooting technique should be taught so that athletes will avoid injury to the arms and be more successful in their attempts. Shooters need good balance; this is attained by bending the knees, evenly distributing body weight on the balls of the feet, and keeping the body straight—not leaning forward or backward. The bent knees supply the power needed to get the ball to the basket. Players who shoot with their arms only rarely make a basket and risk straining their arm muscles.

Passing is another skill that some players pick up haphazardly but which should be learned and practiced with correct form. While waiting for a pass, the hands should be kept up with thumbs together and fingers spread. This will prevent the most common basketball injury—jammed and sprained fingers. Players should also know different types of passes and be prepared to receive them; these include chest pass, bounce pass, baseball pass, and the overhead pass.

Dribbling is a skill that takes a great deal of time and practice to master. For obvious, yet often overlooked, safety reasons, players must learn how to dribble a ball with control and speed with their head *up*. A player who watches the ball is at great risk for collision injuries. Make sure your young players learn to look where they're going while they're dribbling the ball.

Injuries

Basketball was originally conceived as a non-collision sport, but it has evolved into a body-contact activity. Despite rules and regulations that attempt to minimize bodily contact, collisions do happen, making basketball one of the top four sports causing injury. (Basketball comes fourth after football, gymnastics, and wrestling.) Fortunately, serious and fatal injuries are quite rare in this sport. The majority of injuries are caused by falling, overuse of muscle units, and improper technique. The most common injuries include the following.

Abrasions

Basketball players often suffer abrasions and floor burns (page 273) when they fall on the hard wood floor while running.

Ankle Injuries

Ankle injuries account for more time lost from basketball practice and games than any other injury. Ankles are most commonly injured when a player's foot accidentally lands on an opponent's foot while running or coming down from a rebound.

Finger Injuries

Jammed (page 238) or sprained (page 259) fingers commonly occur on the basketball court when players incorrectly catch a pass with the tips of their fingers.

Knee Injuries

Acute knee injuries are rare in this sport. When they do happen it's usually the result of a player falling down on another athlete's leg, or of a player coming down off balance from a jump or rebound.

The chronic "jumper's knee" is commonly found in basketball players, This painful problem is caused by a partial tear in the tendon at the front of the knee joint. It almost always affects the jump leg—in right-handed athletes it affects the left leg; in left-handed players it affects the right leg. Repeated stress on the tendon may cause a microscopic tear that is initially insignificant and so the athlete continues to play. This aggravates the healing process and painful scarring results.

Another overuse injury which can affect basketball players is Osgood-Schlatter's disease (page 258). This inflammation of the knee is caused by repeated small tears at the point of ligament and tendon attachment to the upper tibial bone.

Leg and Foot Injuries

The running, jumping, and rebounding that make up the bulk of basketball activity is hard on the legs and feet. Stress fractures (page 237), shin splints (page 239), and Achilles tendon ruptures (page 282) are most common injuries. An athlete can reduce the risk of leg and foot injury with a pre-season conditioning program of progressive running on hard surfaces to simulate the hard basketball court.

Skin Injuries

Blisters and calluses (page 243) on the feet are the curse of basketball players at the start of the season. Constant stopping, starting, and pivoting make it difficult to avoid these problems, but athletes can reduce their frequency and severity by using properly fitting basketball shoes, two pairs of socks, and bandages in sensitive areas.

Players who have contagious skin conditions such as herpes simplex or impetigo (page 271) should be seen by a physician before they are allowed to continue participation in this sport where there is a maximum amount of exposed body skin as well as on-going bodily contact. All players should be discouraged from sharing towels on the sidelines or in the locker rooms.

Wrist Injuries

Fractured (page 235) and sprained (page 259) wrists are most often the result of falling on an outstretched hand. The wrist is particularly vulnerable to injury when the player falls from a jump position in the air while rebounding or shooting.

Conditioning

The sport of basketball is physically demanding in its continuous and varied pace. The running, stopping, starting, jumping, shooting, throwing requirements of the game put great stress on an unconditioned body. The following suggestions will help your athlete stay injury free and at the same time improve his or her ability to play the game:

flexibility (page 67): Begin each practice and game by stretching the following muscles: shoulder, upper arms, calves, back, groin, and sides. Place special emphasis on the Achilles tendon.

agility (page 71): The footwork drills taught at basketball practices as well as the drills in Chapter Three will develop an athlete's agility skills. Running backwards is also an effective way to teach the body balance and coordination while mimicking the moves of the game.

speed (page 71); Basketball players need to develop their anaerobic capacity. They can do this by running sprints the length of a basketball court. After each sprint, they should rest and recover before running again.

cardiovascular endurance (page 72): Tired players are more easily injured than energetic ones. (They are also more quickly defeated.) Distance running will build the endurance needed to run up and down the court and it will also build the strong legs needed for rebounding and getting off on fast breaks.

strength (page 72): Coaches have found that basketball players who are involved in strength training are less liable to injury and are able to jump higher, run harder without tiring, and pass and rebound better than those who are not. Strength training of the following body parts are most helpful to basketball players: hands, wrists, ankles, arms, legs, knees.

The use of ankle weights during workout to promote the ability to jump and to give the athlete a sense of increased agility should be discouraged until late adolescence. The incidence of "jumper's knee" and Osgood-Schlatter's disease is much higher in skeletally immature players who use these weights.

Basketball demands a great deal from its players. It also gives back a great deal in enjoyment and physical conditioning. Despite the relatively high rate of injuries sustained while playing this sport, you can help ensure a positive and healthy season for your young athlete by monitoring the quality of the equipment, the skill instruction segment of practice sessions, and the implementation of a thorough and on-going conditioning program.

8

■■■■■

Football

Football is a collision sport, and every injury mentioned in this book may be incurred while playing it. If your sons play football, you must understand that the risk of injury is high. At the same time you should know that many injuries common to this sport are preventable. Careful monitoring of safety equipment, practices, and body conditioning can substantially reduce your athlete's risk of sustaining serious injury.

Equipment

All athletes playing on organized football teams are issued safety equipment. Don't assume that whatever they receive is exactly what they need to protect them from injury. The following section will tell you how to check three important safety factors of the equipment: 1) the quality, 2) the fit, and 3) the off-season and in-season maintenance.

Standard Equipment

Helmet and Face Guard

* Because the overwhelming majority of football players are male, we will use the pronoun "he" throughout this chapter.

139

All helmets must bear the NOCSAE seal. This certifies that the helmet has been approved for use by the National Operating Committee on Standards for Athletic Equipment. Some noncertified and less expensive helmets carry labels that boast "Authentic Pro." These are nothing more than toys and will not protect an athlete's head from injury. Do not allow your athlete to play football unless he is wearing a NOCSAE helmet.

The face guards attached to helmets come in a variety of styles. Some have one bar across the face; some have two. Some add a vertical midline bar. Make sure, whichever style your son uses, that the bar does not block his vision. If it does, the helmet does not fit him properly.

All helmets come with a chinstrap. Make sure your son knows that he can not play unless it is snapped across his chin. It is not uncommon for athletes to release the strap while standing on the sidelines, then rush in to play, forgetting to restrap it.

All helmets must be reconditioned, tested, and recertified every year. Make sure you check the NOCSAE seal on the helmet for a certification date, and that your son's football league sends the helmets to a professional sporting goods reconditioner. During the season, teach your son to check for cracks in the shell, and if it is a suspension-type helmet that secures the head with an internal web of straps, instruct him not to untie the knot that controls the web tension once the helmet has been fitted. (If possible, suspension helmets should be replaced with helmets that are filled with air or a combination of air and glycerin. These give a more custom fit and can better absorb the shock of impact.)

Football helmets must fit properly. Even the best equipment will cause injuries rather than prevent them if it is not the right size. If your son's team has an athletic trainer, that person will personally size, distribute, and examine all equipment. Without the benefit of a trainer, the coaches should know how to fit equipment properly. If that isn't the case, you can call your local college athletic department or hospital sports clinic and ask if someone will examine your son's football equipment. If that isn't possible you can follow these guidelines:

1. Place the helmet on the head by putting thumbs in the earholes and tilting the head backwards while you pull down.
2. If it is an air helmet, put it on without air and inflate the outer air pockets with five to seven pumps. (Air pressure should be monitored throughout the season.)
3. With the helmet on, do the following:

- Adjust the chinstrap so that it is snug, with equal tension on both sides.
- Make sure the earholes are over the ear canals or slightly above them, never below them.
- Make sure there are two or three finger widths between the nose tip and the face mask.
- Make sure there are two finger widths between the eyebrow and the beginning of the helmet.
- Make sure the jaw pads are snug.
- Tell your son to hold his head still while you alternately apply rotational and up-and-down force. There should not be much play in the movement; the boy's skin should move with the helmet. The pressure should be on the forehead, not on the eyebrow.
- Interlock your fingers and press down on the top of the helmet. The pressure should be on the crown of the head, not the back or front.

Shoes

According to statistical studies, the safest football shoe is a high-top with short rubber cleats. Unfortunately, many athletes dislike wearing high-tops for football because they are not as popular as the lower cut shoes. When shopping for shoes, however, keep this safety fact in mind and remember that the shorter the cleat the better. When the shoe plants too firmly into the ground the athlete is at risk for a knee injury. Youth-league players should consider playing in well-tractioned sneakers.

Any style or color football shoe must be well fitted, with ample toe room that allows the athlete to wear a second pair of socks for added cushioning. It should also have a well-molded longitudinal arch that gives the foot proper support and the player should always carefully and completely lace the shoe. Make a habit of spraying the shoes with an anti-fungal spray or powder to keep the growth of fungus (and odor) under control; fungus and moisture can eventually cause athlete's foot. Often during the football season shoes become wet and mud-soaked. Because they should dry out completely before being worn at the next game or practice, it is best to buy your athlete two pairs.

If a football player has an ankle problem, the coach or trainer should consider taping the ankle over the shoe and sock to add optimal support. If your athlete wears any type of foot orthotic, the football shoe should have a removable support so that the orthotic can fit firmly and securely on the floor of the shoe. Competitors who play on astroturf will need shorter rubber cleats or even sneakers.

Shoulder Pads

The shoulder pads should not be worn, frayed, or in any other way appear neglected. They should also fit properly: pads which are too large or too small leave the shoulder vulnerable to bruises or separations; if they are too tight in the neck area they can cause a pinched nerve, and if they are too large they do not protect the neck area properly.

Special shoulder pads have been developed specifically for athletes who have had shoulder injuries. Although they are quite a bit more expensive than standard ones, if your athlete is returning to play and you're worried about a re-injury, you should ask the coach to locate and obtain a pair of these ultra-protective pads.

Girdle and Pad Set

All players must wear a girdle that has protective pads over the hip areas and the tailbone.

Thigh Pads

The thigh pads fit into pockets in the player's pants. They protect the thighs from impact bruises.

Knee Pads

Knee pads also fit into pockets in the player's pants. They protect the knees from abrasions and offer some buffer against impact.

Some young players remove the thigh and knee pads because they've seen professional players (especially kickers and wide receivers) remove them to increase their agility and speed. Do not let your sons play without these pads. Even young kickers, who do not wear knee pads, are often sent in to play another position on a moment's notice; make sure they are always well protected.

Mouth Guards

All players *must* wear mouth guards. Some are stock items that are identical in shape and form; others are made of soft plastic that mold to the player's mouth and teeth formation. Make sure that your athlete always wears his mouth guard, does not alter it in any way, and does not use anyone else's.

Athletic Supporter and Cup

The athletic supporter *and* cup are required equipment for players of all ages.

Knee Braces

Some leagues require their players to wear knee braces; others do not. There is controversy over their use because in some instances they offer protection, while in others serve no purpose and encumber the player. The latest studies by the American Academy of Sports Medicine indicate that preventive knee bracing does not seem to prevent knee injuries.

The only kind of knee braces that need to be worn on the football field for preventive purposes are functional ones that are worn to help stabilize a knee that has had a previous injury. Customized braces that are professionally fit to the athlete are the only kind that have been shown to effectively prevent further injury during athletic competition. Although these braces can not completely immobilize the knee, their goal is to prevent significant joint displacement in direct athletic competition. The brace must have both inner and outer (medial and lateral) support as well as straps on the front of the brace that cross the knee joint. The braces should allow full range of motion, especially flexion, without discomfort.

Optional Equipment

Neck Collar

A neck collar is frequently used to help ease the impact on the cervical spine that might occur after contact with another player. The collars do not prevent all whiplash-type injuries, however, especially side-to-side flexion-rotation injuries. An athlete who has had several burners (see page 276) should not use a collar in place of being completely healed before returning to play.

Rib Pads

Rib pads protect the ribs, the kidneys, the liver, and the surrounding mid-area.

Forearm Pads and Elbow Pads

Forearm and elbow pads give protection to these otherwise completely exposed areas.

Hand Pads

Hand and forearm pads are often used by linemen to allow full use of the hands and arms in blocking. These pads are also useful in rehabilitation because they restrict movement in the wrist, elbow, and fingers, and prevent strain to injured joints. Some players, however, have found that the forearm and hand pads also give them greater freedom to use these body parts as weapons. This offensive use of protective equipment should be discouraged.

Gloves

Gloves should be worn by all players (especially linemen) to protect the fingers and hands from the cold and from the multiple scrapes and injuries that can lead to skin and joint infections.

Shock Absorbers

Shock absorbers are rubber paddings worn under the shoulder pads for additional protection. They are usually worn by running backs because these players are most likely to be tackled from the front.

Practice

The condition of the playing area is a factor in calculating the risk of injury while playing football. When you watch a practice, check the playing field for these conditions.

- An unkept, uneven, irregular, rocky, or littered playing surface is extremely hazardous and likely to cause ankle and lower leg injuries.
- Goalposts must be padded.
- The field should have adequate room beyond the endlines so that athletes don't collide with the fences and walls around the stadium.
- Emergency equipment such as bite blades, airway holders, ambu bags, spineboards, or stretchers should be immediately available. Medical personnel and access to ambulances should also be made available during every game. A telephone must be on the field for emergency communication. This is especially important (yet often overlooked) on practice fields, where the trainer, team doctor, and emergency medical teams who are usually close by during weekend games are absent. Car phones, citizen-band radios, and walkie-talkies are useful as backup means of signaling for help, but make sure that wherever your son plays there is an installed and functioning telephone.

When you observe your son's practice sessions, take some time to watch the coaches in action. As explained in Chapter One, the coaches' experience, attitudes, and playing philosophies are factors that also contribute to the risk of incurring injury; this is especially so in the game of football. Studies have found that injury rates have been higher on youth community football teams coached by untrained and/or uncertified younger men (under age 30) as compared to the same kind of coaches over the age of 40. This may happen because the mature, older coaches have more experience and can more readily recognize potentially injurious situations. It is also believed that coaches who demand hard-hitting practices usually have a higher rate of injury on their teams than those who schedule limited contact activities in between games. In fact, today's high school, college, and professional teams tend to use minimal contact sessions, where the players practice hitting only once a week and often use dummies instead of bodies.

The football practice session should be carefully planned to allow time for body conditioning, instruction, and several different types of drills. The session should always begin with a thorough warm-up period that sufficiently warms and stretches the muscles. This should be followed by proper, gradual, and complete physical conditioning, with special emphasis on neck strengthening to reduce the risk of spinal cord injury. The team might then divide up to learn and practice the skills of specific playing positions.

Practice time should also include group and team drills that run through the proper and safe methods of blocking and tackling. Most serious injuries are caused when players use improper blocking and tackling techniques. Make sure that your son knows the right way to play his position, that he abides by the safety rules, and that his coach enforces them. A few of the most important techniques and rules include the following.

- To be in the proper hitting position for blocking and tackling, players should be on the balls of their feet, with their feet approximately shoulder-width apart. They should have a good bend in the knees and at the waist. Backs should be arched, and heads should be up.
- Players should be taught how to tackle around the opponents' thighs and hips with the head up and off center. This

will help them avoid being hit by the knees of the running offensive player.

- Any type of hand contact around an opponent's head should be discouraged.
- There should be no blocking allowed below the waist.
- Players should never "pile on" a player after a tackle has been made.
- Stick-blocking is illegal. Offensive players can not plant their faces into the shirt numerals at the defensive man's mid-section.
- Players must NEVER use their heads as ramming rods, tackling spears, or butting instruments. There has been a significant drop in football-related fatalities, paralysis, cervical fractures, dislocations, and subluxations since 1976, when a rule change outlawed the use of the head as a primary and initial point of contact when blocking or tackling. One study found that the drop from 20 reported football-related fatalities in 1965 to 4 in 1985 was directly attributable to the rule preventing "spearing" and to the improvements in NOCSAE's standards for helmet safety.[1] Your son has the advantage of new safety rules and equipment. Make sure that he knows and uses both.
- If your son's team practices with machines, such as the gauge or spring-loaded impact machine, be sure their use is *closely* supervised and that the athletes thoroughly warm up before the practice. These machines pose a greater threat of injury than the game of football itself.

You, your football player, and the coaches must also keep a sharp eye out for general physical situations that can increase the risk of injury. Make sure that the players in youth leagues, for example, are carefully matched in size and weight. Athletes should be told that because they are more prone to injury when they are fatigued, they must pay attention to their diet and sleep schedules. With this information in mind, ask them to commit to improving their body condition and taking a rest when they are too tired to continue playing. All players must also consistently meet their bodies' need for water. Your young athlete must make a habit of taking water breaks no matter what the weather, and should increase the frequency of these breaks in warm and hot weather.

Injuries

By its very nature, football is a rough sport. Participants are at greater risk of injury than those in any other organized youth sport program. The injury type and frequency for high school players is different, however, than it is for preadolescents. One recent study has found that the overall injury rate for high school players ranges from 25 to 65 percent (depending how "injury" is defined), while that rate for younger players is lower, at 15 percent.[2] This difference may be the result of attitude, coaching, and physiology. Older players may be more likely than younger players to be overly aggressive and to play with less caution. It's also true that older players become less flexible during growing spurts and are naturally more prone to injury.

Although football players are liable to sustain any injury known to sports medicine, the most commonly incurred include the following:

Trauma to the vertebrae and the resulting trauma to the spinal cord (page 275) most often happens during head-to-head tackling. Players attempting to spear an opponent also risk this kind of injury because spearing involves unnatural flexing of the neck.

Next to spinal cord injuries, knee injuries are the most seriously debilitating injuries affecting football players. When a player makes a sudden change in direction with his foot planted on the playing surface, he may tear cartilage (page 254) or ligamental structures (page 222) with his knee.

If a player twists his knee after a direct blow, he may sustain a growth plate fracture (page 236) or an anterior cruciate ligament injury (page 257). A player should take himself out of the game and an orthopedist should be consulted if a player feels or hears a pop or snap at the moment of contact. In the skeletally immature athlete, these knee injuries frequently result in growth plate injuries because the collateral ligaments (those on the side of the knee) are directly over the area of the growth plate and not above it. Therefore the force of impact is absorbed in this region.

Players who come down on their feet unbalanced may suffer sprained ankles (page 259). Contusions (page 274) to the forearm happen quite frequently during blocking and tackling and therefore forearm pads are recommended. And hand injuries are easily sustained when the hand hits against hard objects such as helmets, face masks, shoulder pads, or is stepped on. These injuries may include lacerations (page 274), puncture wounds (page 275), dislocated fingers (page 234); as stated above, gloves should be worn at all times.

Some football injuries are fatal. Most direct fatalities are caused by improper tackling that injures the head and/or neck. Damage to internal organs has also been known to be fatal. Any athlete who, after contact, notices blood or a color change in his urine, or who complains of pain in the abdomen, upper back, or below the rib cage should be examined by a physician. As a preventive measure, players such as receivers, running backs, and quarterbacks, who are tackled quite often, should wear rib pads. These protect the rib cage and offer some impact cushioning to the kidneys and other vital organs, such as the liver and spleen. A smaller number of fatalities have been caused by heart failure, a fact which emphasizes the need for thorough pre-season physicals (see Chapter Four). Some have reportedly been caused by heat stroke; this is certainly a preventable situation that you, your athlete, and the coaches can prevent by being aware of the causes, signs, and symptoms explained on page 251.

See page 92 for a list of medical conditions that may prohibit participation in football.

Conditioning

Most football injuries occur in the first half of the season when the body is not fully conditioned. Athletes can decrease their risk of injury with overall body conditioning. In addition, emphasis should then be placed on building cardiovascular endurance to eliminate the fatigue factor, and on enhancing muscular strength to help the body withstand the rigorous demands of the sport. Your son's coaches can suggest a thorough training regime. The following will give you an idea of the types of exercises that should be included in the conditioning program:

flexibility (page 67): all leg muscles, shoulders, neck.

agility (page 71)

speed (page 71)

cardiovascular endurance (page 72)

muscular endurance (page 72)

strength (page 72): especially of these body parts: neck, legs, arms, hips, and upper body for offensive linemen.

As noted earlier, football-related fatalities have drastically decreased in recent years. Proper training, instruction, and equipment will continue to keep these numbers low. Well-informed coaches and vigilant parents will keep football one of America's most enjoyable sports.

9

■ ■ ■ ■ ■

Gymnastics

Sterling performances at the past few Olympic games have vaulted the sport of gymnastics into the limelight. Gymnastic clubs have sprung up all over the nation and gymnastic competitions have become highly popular events. Because it takes years of hard practice to develop accomplished skills in this sport, many athletes begin their training between the ages of 5 and 8. At such a young age, and throughout the years of gymnastic training, you have a vital role to play in ensuring the health and safety of your young gymnast. The following information will explain some of the basic safety factors to be considered during gymnastic practices and competitions.

Equipment

Apparatus

Gymnastic apparatus such as the balance beam, the vault, the rings, and so forth are quality pieces of equipment made to withstand the stress of the sport. Although you should expect the instructors to make a habit of checking the equipment for signs of wear, breakage is not a real danger or concern. You should, however, check, on an initial visit to the gym, to see that the equipment is properly secured in its place and that there is ample room between each piece to allow safe approach and dismount. You should also look to be sure the floor and mats are dust and clutter free. If they are not, approach and dismount injuries are bound to happen.

Mats

Safety mats are placed under and alongside apparatus to protect the gymnast from a fall and to cushion the jolt of a dismount. Some gymnastic clubs use crash pads which are very thick and soft landing mats that are especially useful for aerial events.

Chalk

Chalk should be used by all gymnasts who perform on the vault, bars, or rings. It is rubbed on the hands before practicing or performing to prevent slipping due to sweat. Gymnasts should make it a habit to check the apparatus before each practice or performance to be sure there is no chalk build-up that will injure their hands and affect their ability to perform their stunt safely. Chalk build-up can be removed with a damp rag or with sandpaper.

Rosin

Rosin should be used on the soles of the footwear to prevent slipping in events that require a running approach and also in the floor exercise and on the balance beam.

Handguards

Handguards fit over the middle two fingers on both hands (some have three finger holes) and are fastened around the wrists with straps. They help to protect the hands from blisters and abrasions and give the gymnast a better grip during events on the bars and rings.

Spotting Belts

Spotting belts support gymnasts in the air while they practice new routines and they protect them from crash landings. These belts are connected to a series of ropes and pulleys that are attached to the ceiling and controlled by the coach.

Shoes

Gymnasts generally wear lightweight slippers made of soft leather with rubberized, non-slip soles. Some prefer a half-shoe which covers only the front of the foot and leaves the heel bare; it is attached around the back of the ankle with an elastic. Others wear socks or nylon stockings, but this should be discouraged for any event that requires good footing, such as the balance beam, floor exercise, and vault.

Clothing

Although each gymnastic club will set its own standards for dress during practice and competition, make sure that your child has a good warm-up sweatsuit to wear when he or she is not performing. This is especially important during competitions; while gymnasts wait for their turn to compete, their muscles cool off after their warm-up exercises and after each performance. Remember—warm muscles are less prone to injury.

Practice

General

Practice sessions must always be supervised by a knowledge-able coach. Gymnastics is not a sport that can be picked up on one's own. All gymnasts must learn proper technique right from the very beginning. This will help prevent them from building bad habits that are difficult to break and that become dangerous as the degree of difficulty increases.

Your child should never attempt to learn a new gymnastic stunt unless a *trained* spotter is present. A professional knows how to support a gymnast and guide the movements to ensure safe completion of the stunt. He or she also knows how to properly "catch" a gymnast who falls. A teammate who stands by "in case someone falls" is not good enough. Once a stunt has been learned and is well practiced, gymnasts may spot each other, but never during the learning stages.

Practice sessions often include trampoline work. Although not a competitive event in itself, trampolines are used to train young gymnasts and to practice body movement and control. Make sure your young athlete knows that, like all other pieces of apparatus, the trampoline is not a toy. Most cervical spinal injuries in gymnastics have been sustained on the trampoline and mini-trampoline. The risk to novice athletes is highlighted by European literature which details the fact that neurologic injuries have been sustained even by expert gymnasts during trampoline workouts. (It has been found that the somersault is the maneuver with the highest potential for serious injury.) The Committee on Accident and Poison Prevention of the American Academy of Pediatrics has issued a policy statement recommending that trampolines be banned from use as part of the physical educational program in grammar schools, high schools, and colleges and also that it be abolished as a competitive sport. Obviously, in gymnastics, trampolines should be used only when highly trained personnel, who have been instructed in all aspects of trampoline safety, are present.

In general, the sport of gymnastics demands a great deal from the body. Thorough warm-ups before every practice and competition are an absolute must if athletes are to avoid injury. In addition, you should make sure that your young athlete follows these general rules at all practices:

- Never practice alone.
- Make sure there are plenty of safety mats under every piece of equipment.

- Make sure the floors and performance surfaces are dust free and uncluttered.
- Remove all jewelry and watches. Tie back long hair. In even the most basic stunts, jewelry and long hair are cumbersome, distracting, and dangerous.
- Never chew gum or eat anything during a training or performance period.

Specific

Practice sessions must be specifically geared to the needs of gymnasts performing particular events. The following will give you an overview of the kinds of safety features to look for when your athlete is performing each kind of gymnastic stunt.

Balance Beam

The balance beam is a girls' event. Each routine consists of a mount, combinations of movements on the beam, and a dismount. For judging purposes the routines should present a picture of confidence, sureness, and control, as well as elegance and grace.

Beginners should practice all stunts in a straight line on the gym floor. They can then advance to a low beam that is just inches off the floor. When they feel confident, then they can try the stunts on the high balance beam. Once your daughter advances to the beam, you should make sure that there are ample safety mats under and around the beam, several feet available on both sides of the beam for dismounts and falls, and a trained spotter alongside the beam.

Conditioning

Athletes training on the balance beam need to develop the following body parts:

flexibility (page 67): arms, groin, hips and hamstrings.

agility (page 71)

strength (page 72): all leg and upper body muscles, lower back to withstand jolt of dismount.

Vault

Vaulting is an event performed by both male and female gymnasts. Female vaulting is a bit different in that the horse is approached from the width side and it is slightly lower in height. Whether male or female, your young athlete should begin vaulting with the horse set as low as possible and gradually increase the height as skill and confidence develops. Before attempting a jump, vaulters must first learn proper running approach and the technique of taking off from both feet. They must also learn how to push downward with their hands when passing over the horse. A double thickness of mats should be placed on the landing side of the horse.

Conditioning

Gymnasts performing on the vault should condition the following body parts:

flexibility (page 67): arms, shoulders, wrists, hips.
strength (page 72): shoulders, upper arms, hands, wrists.

Bars

Female gymnasts perform on the uneven parallel bars; male gymnasts perform on the even parallel bars and the high bar. Safety features during training for these events are similar. These athletes need ample matting under the bars and trained spotters at their side. The beginner should start with the bars lowered as far as possible and progress in height and difficulty of stunt as skill level gradually develops. Bar athletes should wear handguards and use chalk on their hands. They should also make sure the bar is clean of chalk. They should learn how to grasp the bar properly and should limit their learning workouts to short periods so as to avoid painful and debilitating blisters and skin tears.

Conditioning

Athletes training on the bars should condition the following body parts:
   flexibility (page 67): shoulders, arms, groin, and hamstrings.
   agility (page 71)
   strength (page 72): shoulders, upper arms, chest, back, wrists, and hands.

Rings

Ring performances require exceptional arm and chest strength and are therefore performed solely by male gymnasts. Because the rings are in a fixed position they can not be moved around the gym, and so all other equipment and gymnasts should be moved away from the ring area when they are in use. Rings require very little floor area, with a 5' × 10' safety mat offering ample protection. Beginners should practice on rings that are lowered to approximately shoulder height. As skill level progresses, the rings may slowly be elevated to the regulation competitive height of about eight feet from the floor. A trained spotter should stand to one side of the gymnast the entire time a stunt is being attempted. The instructor should help the beginning gymnast through the stunts and be positioned to catch him in case of a slip or fall.

Conditioning

Gymnasts will enhance their work on the rings by conditioning the following body parts:
   flexibility (page 67): Shoulder flexibility is especially important when the gymnast is performing stunts that involve twisting and turning of the arms while the joint is extended.

strength (page 72): arms, shoulders, chest, and hands.

Floor Exercise

The floor exercise is performed by male and female gymnasts alike. The females' event is different from the males' in that it is performed to music and emphasizes graceful ballet-like movements. The males' event is performed without music and emphasizes movements of power and strength. For both, the floor exercise offers an opportunity for creative and imaginative input in developing a routine that consists of jumps, turns, spins, balancing and agility movements, and tumbling sequences.

Beginning gymnasts should learn the floor exercise movements in carefully plotted sequences. As your child learns the movements that include split, walkover, handstand, forward roll, cartwheel, round-off, handspring, and back flip, an instructor/spotter should always be close by to guide the body through the movements and catch the gymnast if he or she should fall. All practices and performances should be executed on safety mats.

Your daughters may enjoy training for an event that was introduced at the 1984 Olympic games. Rhythmic gymnastics is like a floor exercise, but it is performed on a carpet or linoleum floor and the girls hold and manipulate hand apparatuses such as hoops, balls, ropes, clubs, and ribbons. These add a degree of difficulty to the stunts as well as color and drama.

Conditioning

Athletes who perform floor exercises use a wide array of body moves and physical stunts. Their conditioning program should be one that is generalized to develop overall flexibility (page

67), cardiovascular endurance (page 72), and strength (page 72).

Injuries

As in most sports, gymnastic injuries fall into two categories: acute trauma injuries and overuse or repetitive stress injuries. The first type of injury is caused by sudden acute traumas that happen when, for example, an athlete falls off the balance beam, or bangs the body into the uneven parallel bar, or stumbles in a tumbling routine. Common acute injuries sustained by gymnasts include sprains (page 259), strains (page 268), fractures (page 235), and dislocations (page 234) of the toes, feet, ankles, elbows, shoulders, and wrists. (Ankle sprains are perhaps the most common single injury in gymnastics.) Lack of confidence, skill, and conditioning increase the risk of sudden accident and so the majority of acute trauma injuries are found in the less skilled gymnasts. Beginners are also more likely than advanced gymnasts to suffer the discomforts of hand blisters (page 243) and muscle contusions (page 264).

Most acute injuries sustained by gymnasts are preventable. Studies have found that these injuries can be greatly reduced in number when gymnasts are trained in proper technique and progress gradually through the skill levels. Thick floor mats and attentive spotters will also reduce the risk of incurring these injuries.

The second type of injury develops gradually and is caused by overuse or repetitive stresses on the musculoskeletal system. These will present themselves when, for example, gymnasts spend years jarring their body in dismounts, or twisting their wrists and shoulders in bar and ring exercises. The cumulative effect of this jarring and twisting is found primarily in the advanced gymnast because symptoms occur only after extended periods of stress on the muscles, tendons, or bones. The increase in the number of children training at age 4 and 5 and continuing training for the following 10 years or so has increased the number of overuse and stress injuries being treated by physicians today. Most commonly these injuries affect the wrist, the knee, the ankle and foot, and the spine.

Wrist injuries are usually of two kinds: 1) wrist synovitis (page 279) and 2) stress fractures (page 237) of the carpal bones in the wrist.

Common knee injuries include: 1) chrondromalacia petella (page 255), 2) tendonitis (page 258), 3) Osgood Schlatter's disease (page 258), 4) epiphyseal plate injuries (page 236) of the proximal tibia.

Several studies have found the ankle and foot to be the body area most commonly injured by gymnasts. Stress and overuse injuries include: 1) ankle synovitis (page 279), which may be caused by improper dismount, 2) tenosynovitis (page 282), and 3) Achilles tendonitis (page 281), which results from the impact of repetitive dismount and from tumbling exercises.

Hyperextension, or repetitive arching of the back, (especially during dismount) may result in a fatigue fracture (page 237) of the spine. Sometimes athletes don't know they have this injury because it may take months before the fracture and surrounding inflammation become obvious. If your child complains of back pain (especially with hyperextension of the lower back) a thorough spinal evaluation should be undertaken.

The above should not be taken to imply that you should limit or forbid gymnastic training at an early age, but it does mean that to raise a healthy athlete you should know that this kind of spinal trauma can occur, and the risk of occurrence can be reduced with proper instruction by trained gymnastic coaches and with a limitation on the number of daily dismounts practiced. If your child begins gymnastic instruction at an early age and you expect that he or she will continue serious training for another 8 to 10 years, then you should also know how to assure early detection of spinal stress fractures. Serious students should begin gymnastic training with a physical examination that includes a thorough back exam.

See page 92 for a list of medical conditions that may prohibit participation in gymnastics.

Gymnastics is a sport that, perhaps more than any other, offers untold personal satisfaction in achievement through skill progression. It also, however, subjects the growing musculoskeletal system to a variety of acute injuries and stresses that the body may not be able to withstand. Your awareness of the specific areas of body stress, and your monitoring of preventive strategies through skilled coaching, thorough conditioning, and prompt treatment of problems will go a long way to ensuring continued safe enjoyment of this graceful, highly skilled, and personally rewarding sport.

10

■ ■ ■ ■ ■

Soccer

A s a popular sport in 135 countries, soccer is played by more people than any other sport in the world. In the United States alone, over 1.88 million players under the age of 19 enjoy this sport, which is an excellent body conditioner and requires a minimum of equipment and expense. Although soccer injuries are reported to be only one-fifth as frequent as and less severe than injuries sustained in American football, soccer players are still prone to lower extremity injuries.[1] The following information will help you reduce the number and severity of these injuries through proper monitoring of equipment, practices, and conditioning regimes.

Equipment

Shoes

The soccer shoe is a cleated one that should give support and as much contact with the ground as possible. Multi-cleated shoes that have short, rubber cleats over the entire foot area are most often recommended by soccer coaches.

Shoes that have only a few cleats on the bottom (which are usually longer than average size) are fine for playing on a soft or wet surface, but younger girls and boys who don't

weigh enough to push the cleats into harder ground may find
that the shoes with fewer cleats do not give them as much
support as the multi-cleated shoes. In fact, young players
might do better to wear a good running shoe without cleats
that gives them proper arch support.

It is very important for shoes to fit properly. Shoes that
are too small or too big can cause injury to the back, hip,
or knee areas.

The soccer shoe must also be comfortable. Most playing
and practice time is spent running and so the shoe must give
comfortable support and be as lightweight as possible. New
shoes must be well broken-in before active play to avoid
blisters. Greasing socks with Vaseline® can also help to prevent foot blisters.

Shin Guards

In some leagues shin guards are required equipment, in others
they are optional. Make sure that your young athlete wears
them. Because the majority of soccer injuries are to the lower
extremities, shin guards are the first line of injury prevention
in the game of soccer.

A recent study has found that failure to wear shin guards
markedly increased the proportion of leg injuries. Of all
injured players in this study who wore shin guards, only 2.2
percent sustained an injury to a leg. Of all players documented
as not wearing shin guards at the time of injury, 10.5 percent
had leg injuries.[2]

Shin guards are made in many styles and of varying quality.
The most ineffective are those that are made of thin plastic
and slide inside the sock. These often fall out or move around
inside the sock (even when secured with velcro) and leave
the leg unprotected. Better ones cover the entire shin (some
bend around the entire leg) and give some protection and
support to the ankle. These are sewn inside the sock or are
secured with a foot stirrup. Today, for maximum protection,

shin guards even come with a protective air cushion under the outer plastic layer.

Goalie Equipment

In addition to shin guards, the goalie should wear the following protective garb:

- goalie pants with hip pads.
- goalie shirts with elbow pads; some also have shoulder pads.
- knee pads.
- goalie gloves with a piece of hard plastic on the outside of the hand.
- helmets—rubber helmets have recently become optional goalie equipment; in the near future the use of these helmets may become more commonplace.
- Although not required, goalies should wear protective eye wear, as explained in Chapter Four.

Ball

Soccer balls come in three sizes: size 3 for the youngest players, size 4 for middle-league players, and size 5 for players of 12 years and older. A smaller ball gives younger players better control and reduces the risk of injury posed by larger and harder balls. If your child's youth league is playing with size 5 balls, you should ask the league to invest in the appropriate smaller-sized ones, and in the interim slightly deflate the larger ball to give the kids better control, more play opportunity, and reduce their risk of injury.

Playing Field

Check to be sure the soccer field is free of broken glass, loose rocks, and debris. If possible in outdoor soccer, choose a grass field over a hard surface field. Grass offers a cushioned running surface which reduces the chances of injury from falls; it also offers better footing and absorbs the impact on the body of running and jumping.

Goalposts

Nationwide, during the eight-year period from 1973 through 1980, six children in the age group 5 to 14 died while playing soccer. Four of these deaths occurred when goalposts fell on the players.[3] While this number of fatalities is relatively minimal in the arena of sports play, it is still an indication that the security of the goalposts must be checked periodically.

Practices

All practices should begin with warm-up drills and all players should be actively involved.

As the first rule of soccer, players must learn to look where they're going while playing the ball. Half of all soccer injuries result from player collisions and in the past serious injuries have resulted when players ran into goalposts.

Players should be instructed on the proper footwork (using both feet) and body movements of these techniques:

- controlling
- passing
- dribbling
- heading

Although definitive studies regarding the safety of heading a soccer ball have not been published, concern has recently been raised about the potential for brain injury resulting from this practice. The common occurrence of two inexperienced players attempting to head the ball at the same time can cause head injuries ranging from mild concussions to brain laceration and death. All heading should be discouraged on the pre–high school level.

Even older players need to be carefully coached regarding

the proper way to hit a ball with one's head. A few strategies include:

- Keep eyes open and head up. If a player is looking down, the ball will hit the top of the head incorrectly.
- Look at the ball and let it hit off the forehead.
- Use full body movement to propel the ball forward. Do not try to pass the ball off the head using neck muscles only. Players can absorb the impact of the ball and avoid headaches by remembering this piece of advice—you hit the ball; don't let it hit you.

Injuries

In a study of injuries encountered during participation in a summer soccer camp for youths aged 6 through 17 years, lower extremity injuries accounted for 70.8 percent of all injuries. The findings of this study seem to parallel other studies of the sport. They include:

- Boys most frequently suffer quadricep strains (page 268).
- Girls (who are consistently reported to have a higher incidence of injury than boys) most frequently suffer sprained ankles (page 259).
- There is an abrupt increase in injury incidence near age 14.
- Contact with other players caused the majority of injuries, with 35.2 percent of the players suffering contusions (page 274).
- Non-contact injuries included:
  strains (27.8 percent) page 268
  sprains (19.4 percent) page 259
  fractures(page 235) and dislocations (page 234) accounted for only 2 percent of all injuries.[4]

Overuse injuries are also quite common in soccer. The

running and kicking demands of the sport can inflict recurrent microtrauma to the foot, ankle, knee, or groin. Soccer players commonly suffer from shin splints (page 239), Osgood-Schlatter's (page 258), and Sever's disease (page 238). For this reason these athletes should be well conditioned, and you should watch for the signs of over-training listed on page 65.

If your daughter plays soccer, you may need to be especially vigilant in your efforts to monitor safe sports play. Girls generally sustain more injuries while playing soccer than boys do playing football. This is most likely due to the fact that soccer is one of the few sports in which girls can enjoy truly aggressive play. Although it is an excellent outlet for pent-up energy and frustration, it can also be dangerous.

See page 91 for a list of medical conditions that may prohibit participation in soccer.

Conditioning

Like all athletes, soccer players need general body conditioning, warm-up and cool-down periods, and flexibility training. In addition, jumping rope (page 71) is particularly helpful to soccer players because it improves aerobic capacity, coordination, and the ability to move the feet quickly. Specific to this sport, the athlete should condition for the following:

flexibility (page 67): all leg muscles, hips and neck

agility (page 71)

speed (page 71)

cardiovascular endurance (page 72) This is especially important for halfbacks.

strength (page 72): all leg muscles.

Specifically, to help soccer players better withstand the quick starting, stopping, and changing of direction so vital to the game, athletes should do strength training of the following body parts: ankles, knees, hip joints.

To execute heading the ball safely, high school players

should also strengthen their shoulders and necks. (Pre–high school players should not head the ball.)

Soccer is an indoor, outdoor, fall, and spring sport that is growing in popularity among boys and girls of all ages. Young athletes who play this game enjoy perfecting the skills that improve performance and reduce the risk of injury. They also benefit from the cardiovascular workouts inherent in the game.

11

■■■■■

Tennis

Tennis is a sport that can be played and enjoyed throughout one's lifetime. It is a skilled sport that requires knowledge of proper technique, practice, as well as speed, agility, and muscular and cardiovascular endurance. The following information will help you make sure that your young players reap the benefits of the game and avoid the problems that can sideline them or turn them off completely.

Equipment

Tennis Racquet

Tennis racquets are available in a variety of sizes, styles, weights, and compositions. Some features, such as regular and large racquet heads, can be selected on the basis of personal preference. But there are some features that should be carefully considered before your young athlete chooses his or her racquet. Young players should play with junior racquets that are scaled down in size. The exact age at which a player should switch to an adult racquet is difficult to pinpoint because proper fit depends on the athlete's size and strength, but generally junior racquets are used by prepubescent athletes. These racquets are easier to manage; they give the

170

athlete better control, and are less likely to put undue strain on the wrist and forearm.

The weight of the racquet is another consideration that should be carefully matched to your child's age and needs. In the learning stage, players should use lightweight racquets because they are easier to handle and therefore make it easier to concentrate on proper technique. As players advance in skill, they can move on to slightly heavier racquets as long as they can maintain comfort and control. The heavy racquets that are sometimes used by professional players are generally not appropriate for young athletes.

Be sure the handle grip fits your child's hand. An over-sized grip will make it difficult for players to control the ball and may cause them continually to hit the ball incorrectly. This makes it extremely difficult to use proper technique and will put undue strain on the muscle units of the body. Conversely, a handle that is too small will cause a player to hold the racquet too tightly, which can contribute to the phenomenon known as "tennis elbow." Proper grip fit is generally determined by comfort and ability to manage the racquet, but a basic guideline suggests that when a player grips the racquet, the thumb should meet the first knuckle on the index finger.

The composition of the racquet frame is often a matter of personal choice. You should know, however, that fiberglass and ceramic frames are more flexible than graphite and aluminum ones. Beginning players are often advised to begin with flexible frames and then advance to the stiffer ones that are better able to absorb the stress of hard hitting and therefore put less pressure on the muscle-tendon units of the forearm.

When you purchase a tennis racquet, the string tension you choose will also affect the amount of stress that is put on the arm and elbow. A tightly strung racquet delivers more impact on the ball, but on the player's arm as well. Looser strings take some impact off the ball and they also deliver less stress to the arm muscles. It is not advisable to buy a pre-strung racquet because if the strings have been on the racquet for a long time they will have no tension.

Tennis Balls

Most matches are played with new balls because they are more responsive to the racquet stroke and have more bounce than used balls. During practices, however, teammates will hit for hours with old and/or unpressurized balls that force them to hit the ball harder. That's why proper technique is especially important throughout practice sessions because these older balls cause increased impact and stress on the forearm.

Shoes

Tennis players need shoes specifically made for tennis. "Street-wear" sneakers, running shoes, basketball shoes, aerobic dance shoes, and so on do not give the kind of foot support needed during the stop-and-go action of tennis.

The tennis shoe should be relatively lightweight and well ventilated. It should hold the heel firmly in place and yet allow for ample forefoot room. It should also support the medial arch area as well as give lateral support to control foot movement.

Clothing

In hot weather tennis players should wear clothing that helps them manage the heat. White clothing is best because it reflects the sun away from the body. Cotton material is better able than synthetics to absorb perspiration and allow for sweat evaporation and body cooling. If a player's shirt becomes soaked with perspiration, it should be exchanged for a dry one because wet material can not effectively conduct heat away from the body.

Practice

All practices should begin with ample time for warm-ups. After appropriate stretching (see "flexibility exercises" listed below), tennis warm-ups are sometimes incorporated into workouts that emphasize proper mechanics. To do this, some coaches practice the "20 percent theory" of warming up. They instruct their players to move their feet quickly in place, but to use a slow swing that gradually and effectively warms the muscles involved in play. After ten to fifteen minutes of this skill-practice warm-up, the players are ready for safe participation in active play.

Tennis is a game in which knowledge of proper technique is especially important for enjoyment and competition, as well as for injury prevention. All practices should emphasize the three parts of executing a shot: first, the footwork required to get to the ball and get into position to hit the ball; second, the correct bodily mechanics involved in bringing the racquet back in preparation to hit the ball—the swing stroke itself, and the follow-through arm motion; and third, the use of recovery steps after hitting the ball needed to prepare for the next shot.

These skills can be learned through off-court instruction, by playing the game, and by practicing drill work and patterns. Some coaches find it helpful to create the muscle memory necessary to develop consistency in stroke production by running drills that simulate the proper footwork and stroke without using a ball.

When you watch your athlete practice, make sure that skill instruction and practice are integral parts of the session. Also, check for the routine implementation of safety practice. To prevent falls and sprained ankles, players should frequently clear the balls that clutter the court during active drill work. There should also be plenty of playing space between players. More than two participants in a half-court area invites injury from collision and from being struck with a racquet.

Injuries

Tennis is a non-contact sport and therefore a relatively safe one. Most injuries are caused by overuse of muscle units and are the result of poor conditioning and/or improper technique. Therefore the majority of the following injuries can be prevented with proper conditioning and skill instruction.

Muscle Cramps

Muscles react negatively to fluid loss, fatigue, and tension. In tennis, these factors combine most frequently in heat and high humidity to cause muscle cramps (page 264). Your athlete can prevent the pain and debilitation of muscle cramps by stretching thoroughly before playing and by maintaining fluid intake throughout the playing time.

Shoulder Pain

Tennis players may suffer the pain of tendonitis in the shoulder area (page 281). The discomfort is usually most notable during the act of serving, hitting an overhead shot, or hitting a high backhand stroke. Tendonitis should be suspected if the player experiences pain when executing these shots and yet can hit a forehand or low backhand stroke without soreness.

Muscle strains (page 268) and impingement syndrome (page 252) in the shoulder can be caused by overly aggressive overhand serves. Any feeling of arm numbness or sensation of loose or dislocated shoulder bones should receive professional evaluation promptly.

Tennis Elbow

The most common affliction to strike tennis players is the condition dubbed "tennis elbow" (page 270). This is marked by elbow pain when hitting a backhand shot and is most often experienced by players who play frequently and/or those who use improper technique. To avoid tennis elbow, young players

should be encouraged to use a two-handed backhand technique, keep the wrist firm during the backhand shot, and hit
the ball out in front of the body. The forearm and elbow will
absorb less impact of play if the player uses a larger-head
racquet that is strung at a slightly lower tension and has the
proper grip size.

Ankle Sprains

A tennis player is prone to first- or second-degree ankle sprains
(page 259) because as he or she moves laterally, the foot may
catch and turn in on the ankle. Athletes playing on hard courts
with non-supportive shoes are at increased risk for this injury.
To prevent ankle sprains, gentle, static stretching of the Achilles
tendon must be emphasized in tennis warm-ups.

See page 92 for a list of medical conditions that may prohibit
participation in tennis.

Conditioning

Tennis players need cardiovascular endurance, as well as flexibility, speed, agility, and muscular strength. Even when fatigued, they must be able to hit the ball hard and to run fast
to cover the net as well as the back court. The following
exercises will give your athlete a sport-specific conditioning
regime as well as cross-training exercises for total body conditioning:

flexibility (page 67): The following body parts should be
stretched before and after every tennis session: shoulder and
neck, hips, groin, hamstrings, quadriceps, heel cords, Achilles
tendon.

agility: Tennis players should practice at home the footwork
drills mapped out during tennis sessions. The agility drills on
page 71 will also help them improve balance, coordination,
and quick foot movement.

speed (page 71): The tennis player needs anaerobic bursts

of sudden speed. To simulate the fast and slow run pattern of a game, athletes should practice repeat intervals.

cardiovascular endurance (page 72): A tennis player can increase aerobic capacity through recreational activities such as bicycling, jogging, and swimming.

strength (page 72): Most tennis injuries are caused by overuse trauma to muscle units. Players can decrease the risk of overuse injuries by strengthening the muscles most commonly stressed by the sport. These include: abdomen, shoulders, upper arm, and wrist.

Tennis is a sport that enhances physical development and body fitness. It is played by males and females, both indoors and outdoors, and is popular from elementary school age through to the senior citizen set. If your young athletes play this sport, they are developing positive habits of physical activity that will foster good health for a lifetime.

12

■■■■■

Track and Field

M ost track events trace their origins back to ancient times where they are documented in the records of the earliest Olympic Games. They encompass a variety of running, throwing, and jumping activities. Some emphasize sudden, explosive movements while others focus on endurance capabilities.

Because each track event requires specific equipment, techniques, and conditioning regimes to lower the risk of injury particular to that event, each will be discussed separately in this chapter. The following information about track shoes and daily practices, however, is generally applicable to all track and field athletes.

Equipment

Shoes

Of the several hundred styles of track shoes available to your young athlete, none stands out above the others as best or ideal. Each athlete must take time to find one that is most appropriate for his or her event, is comfortable, and allows room for foot movement. Finding shoes that fit properly and allowing time to break them in completely will help the athlete avoid blisters, calluses, corns, cracked nails, and bleeding under the nail. When you find such a shoe you should purchase two or three pairs. This will enable your young athlete to avoid the injuries caused by having to use a brand new pair that is not broken in when the first pair wears out. This will also give the athlete an immediately available clean, dry pair for meets where inclement weather soaks or damages the original pair.

Although spikes are sometimes worn for track and field events, athletes should begin early season training in "flats" that have superior shock-absorbing capacity. This will reduce the risk of shin splints which occur in early training because the leg muscles aren't yet conditioned to absorb the constant pounding of track activity. Track shoes must not be too stiff. If they do not bend easily at the ball of the foot, the athlete will be forced to "run over" the shoe's end and risk Achilles tendonitis, shin splints, or strains.

The entire inner sole of the shoe should be padded. This can reduce the incidence of midfoot sprains, spurring at the ball of the foot, and bone bruising of the heel. The midfoot should be supported with a slight wedge. Many track and field athletes also find that a raised heel absorbs shock and decreases the risk of straining the Achilles tendon. Proper footwear is an important piece of safety equipment in track and field events. Whichever type and style your child chooses, make sure that it fits properly and gives cushioned support.

Practice

Regardless which track event your athlete participates in, practices that emphasize safety, proper technique, and body conditioning are absolutely necessary to prevent injury in these sports. It's dangerous for anyone to jump into a competitive situation without preparing the body or knowing exactly how to perform the athletic feat. Watch practices to be sure that they begin with warm-ups, that technique and skill instruction (as explained in each section below) is emphasized, that the athletes are taught how to strengthen the body parts stressed by their event and yet are not subjected to over-training.

While observing practice routines, you should also take time to examine the physical environment of the arena. Track athletes are easily injured if the ground is too hard, uneven, littered, rocky, potholed, or in any other way neglected. Also, be sure that your young athlete is using equipment that is of the proper composition, size, and weight for the particular field event (as described below). You would not be overstepping the bounds of positive parental involvement if you called the coaches' attention to dangerous situations and worked with them to improve the playing fields. Teach your children how to examine the environment and equipment for potentially injurious factors. When they are practicing or competing, they should know when to call attention to problems before workouts or competitions begin.

Running Events

Sprinting

Sprinters run at full speed for the entire duration of their event. They depend on fast-twitch muscle fibers (page 52) for this quick burst of explosive energy.

Equipment

Sprinters can wear either standard flat running shoes or spikes with pins on the front half of the shoe. If running on a cedar track, half-inch pins are advisable to prevent slipping. When running on an all-weather track, flat running shoes or spikes with pins no longer than one-quarter inch are appropriate.

Sprinters propel their bodies into quick motion by pushing off from starting blocks. These blocks are pre-set with the front block fixed at a point between 16 and 20 inches behind the starting line. The exact distance is determined by the runner. The rear block is placed approximately 15 inches behind the front one, again depending on the preference of the runner. Your athletes should experiment and make adjustments in these blocks until they fit their individual needs and they can start with comfort and security.

Practices

Sprinters should not begin early season training in spikes or at full speed. They should use supportive and padded running shoes, train on soft surfaces, and allow time for progressive build-up of ability. These athletes must use proper technique to avoid undue stress on their muscle units. They should run with a forward lean, with knees lifting up, and with arms bent and moving forward and back, not side to side. Sprinters can avoid muscle tension (and subsequent soreness) by learning to relax when they run; they should not tighten their arm and upper body muscles, and they should keep the jaw and face muscles loose. It is dangerous for runners to stop abruptly at the finish line; make sure they know to run through the finish and slow down gradually. Also, remind your young athlete that warm muscles will not injure as easily as cold ones, so in cool weather sprinters should keep sweat pants on whenever they are not actually running or competing.

Injuries

Hamstring muscle pulls (page 265) are the most common injury for sprinters. Achilles tendonitis (page 281) and stress fractures (page 237) of the lower leg are also problems for these runners.

Conditioning

Sprinters are prone to leg injuries caused by either lack of proper body conditioning or overuse. These injuries can be greatly reduced in number through the following exercises.

flexibility (page 67): hamstring, Achilles tendon, quadriceps, and hips.

speed (page 71)

strength (page 72): quadricep, hamstring, calf.

Relays

Relay racing involves speed, endurance, and teamwork. It's an event in which two and sometimes four runners run a specific distance and are then relieved by another runner who continues the race.

Practices

Relay runners are sprinters. Therefore, in addition to the following, their practices should include the same drills and skill practices stated above for sprinters. The first relay runner in each race starts from starting blocks. Therefore, just as sprinters do, all relay runners should practice adjusting the blocks to fit their individual needs. Safe relay running requires untiring practice of synchronized baton exchange. Runners should walk through and slowly jog through many practice hand-offs before it is attempted at full speed.

Injuries

The relay runner is prone to the same leg injuries as the sprinter. In addition, however, the baton exchange poses an additional risk of injury. Contusions (page 274) or laceration (page 274) of the hip can happen if the baton misses the open hand of the waiting runner and is then shoved into his or her hip. The batons can also injure the runners' hands if they are not padded. Your athlete can avoid hand punctures and lacerations by checking to be sure there are no sharp edges on the baton. Puncture wounds (page 275), contusion (page 274) to the ankle or calf, or ankle sprain (page 259) can happen if the spiked shoe of the in-coming runner runs over the foot of the waiting runner. Also, lacerations (page 274), jammed fingers (page 238), or dislocated fingers (page 234) can happen from improper exchange of the baton.

Conditioning

The physical demands on a relay runner are the same as those of a sprinter. The conditioning suggestions listed for sprinters should also be practiced by relay runners.

Hurdling

Hurdling is a sprinting event in which the participants run at full speed and then jump over a series of obstacles called hurdles. The hurdler needs the speed of the sprinter as well as the explosive spring action of the jumper.

Equipment

Because of the running speed required in this event, most hurdles wear sprinters' spikes. Newer, specially designed hurdlers' shoes have raised heels and spikes in the front only. This encourages the hurdler to land on the balls of the feet and it pads the heel if the athlete should land incorrectly.

The hurdle itself should be routinely examined for any sharp edges or broken pieces of aluminum which can make it less stable and likely to cause injury.

Practice

During practice sessions the standard routine must be altered for novice hurdlers. Beginners should always practice on grass to decrease the number of abrasions and injuries caused by falling on hard surfaces. Also, soft-top hurdles should be used and athletes should wear sponge rubber protectors on their heels, ankles, and knees.

All hurdlers must learn how to land properly. Athletes

should land on the balls of their feet because landing flat-footed or on the heel will cause foot injuries. Participants who persistently land on their heels should wear heel cups while training to prevent heel bruising.

Emphasizing technique during practice will also reduce the risk of injury in this event. Hurdlers should be taught to keep their arms out in front of the body while attempting a jump. Arms that are stretched straight out to the side will slow forward momentum and this can cause the trailing leg or ankle to hit the hurdle. These athletes must keep their eyes forward at all times because looking back shortens their stride, decreases their forward momentum, and puts them at risk for injury.

Sometimes, to save practice time and energy, hurdlers run through a series of hurdles and then turn around and run through them again from the end of the course back to the beginning. This is a very dangerous practice that puts the hurdler at increased risk for injury because hurdles are designed to tip over only from front to back. Make sure your young hurdler knows why hurdles must be approached only from the front.

Injuries

Hurdlers are at risk for the same kinds of running injuries common to sprinters, with the additional risk of muscle pulls and fractures caused by the degree of stretch needed to clear the hurdle and the danger of hitting the hurdle. Most common injuries include hamstring strain (page 268), groin pull (page 265), and separation of the hip muscles from their pelvic attachment.

Conditioning

Because hurdlers are sprinters who must jump imposed barriers, their conditioning is the same as that for a sprinter (page 180) with special emphasis on the flexibility training and the addition of hip flexibility exercises (page 69).

Distance Running

Distance running includes several kinds of events. Distance running may encompass courses from 400 meters to two-, three-, or six-mile runs. Marathons are run on courses over 25 miles in length (and should not be attempted by athletes on the pre-high school level of competition.) Because of the distances involved, these races place demands on the athlete's slow-twitch muscle fibers and aerobic capacity.

Equipment

The distance runner needs a comfortable and supportive shoe. It must be well padded to absorb repetitive shock. It should have a raised heel to encourage forward lean, support at the midfoot to give the foot needed strength, and the ball area of the shoe must be flexible to allow for ease of push-off. The shoe must be well broken-in before competition.

Practice

Distance running requires exceptional aerobic capabilities. Therefore, practices should emphasize aerobic activities. But keep in mind that the point at which a runner will fatigue varies with each individual. Practices must, therefore, be individualized to each athlete's needs. These competitors should vary their style to run long distances at less than race pace, shorter distances at race pace, and even shorter distances at faster than race pace. Because long-distance running can be a lonely sport, runners should occasionally vary their route, routine, and practice exercises to avoid burnout from boredom. The use of headphones to relieve this boredom should be prohibited in all sports such as running that require prolonged concentration. They significantly dull the athlete's perception of surroundings and mask impending danger of collision with another athlete or inanimate objects such as cars.

Also, to prevent injury track athletes need to learn the mechanics of distance running. In brief:

1. Runners should land on the balls of the foot and rock to the heel.

2. Runners should use short strides because if the stride is too long the foot lands in front of the center of gravity. This causes the runner to slow the pace and work against the natural forward movement.

3. Hands should be carried above the wrists and arms should swing in a relaxed manner from the side to midline of the body. Excessive swinging and pumping motions are counter-productive.

Injuries

Most commonly, the injuries sustained by distance runners are caused by poor body conditioning, lack of proper supervision, or over-training. Shin splints (page 239) and leg stress fractures (page 237) occur most frequently in the early part of the season before the shock-absorbing abilities of the legs are well-established. Fatigue of the diaphram muscles may cause a runner to feel cramps (page 264) in his or her side. This happens when the body is not properly conditioned or when the runner is trying to perform above his or her capability level. If this happens, the runner must decrease the pace or stop completely to allow the body's circulation to catch up to the demands for energy. Once a runner is fatigued, the risk of injury increases because he or she will change the even and relaxed running stride and the use of efficient foot propulsion. Coaches must watch for signs of fatigue and runners must be taught how to recognize their fatigue limit (page 65). Heat exhaustion (page 249) and heat stroke (page 251) are enemies of distance runners. Both, however, are easily preventable and coaches and runners must stay alert to their warning signs.

Long-distance runners usually experience some pain of muscle fatigue while running; it's part of the sport. Unfortunately, this acceptance of pain makes them prone to overuse injuries. Long-distance runners tend to run even when injured, return to the sport before injuries are fully rehabilitated, and practice to the point of over-training. Help your young long-distance runner understand the difference between the expected pain of mild muscle fatigue and the pain signals of injury. If the pain continues even after a period of rest, the athlete has suffered an injury; depending on the type and location of the pain, continued rest or medical care is a must to avoid further injury to the affected area.

Conditioning

Aerobic conditioning for distance running is the single most important factor in injury prevention in this sport. However, aerobic conditioning that increases the cardiovascular endurance capabilities of an athlete must follow the rules of adaption and progression explained in Chapter Three. Runners must never attempt to run at full steam for the full length of the course without proper and gradual conditioning. A precipitous increase in distance will lead to fatigue caused by a build-up of lactic acid (see Chapter Three) and is associated with shin splints (page 239) and stress fractures (page 237). Off-season conditioning programs that strive to maintain aerobic capabilities are especially useful to the distance runner. During the season the following conditioning suggestions should be incorporated into each practice:

- Before running distances, runners need to warm up the oxygen-dependent slow-twitch muscle fibers. That's why their warm-up exercises need to be of longer duration than that of the sprinters.

• After completing a distance course, runners need to cool-down by continuing to jog a bit further. This will prevent future bouts with muscle fatigue.
• Running up and down hills is an efficient way to increase aerobic capacity, improve cardiac fitness, and strengthen leg muscles.
• Distance runners should also train for flexibility (page 67), cardiovascular endurance (page 72), and muscular endurance (page 72).

Throwing Events

Throwing events involve complex skills that maximize the force of momentum and propulsion. Each event requires special equipment, technique training, and conditioning. However, the safety rules boxed on following page apply to all throwing events on all levels of play. Make sure that your child's coaches enforce these rules that protect the participant, his or her teammates, and spectators as well.

Shot-Put

Shot-putting is a power event involving driving action of the legs and hips, coupled with the explosive thrusting action of the arm. The objective of this event is to gain enough momentum within the restrictions of a seven-foot circle to throw a weighted ball the farthest distance possible.

Equipment

Shot-putters usually wear a shoe with a smooth sole that allows them to glide across the circle. There are shoes specially designed for this event.

Shots are made of iron, bronze, or brass with a lead center. The weight of this sphere depends on the age and sex of the athlete: high school boys use a 12-pound ball, high school

GENERAL SAFETY RULES
FOR ALL THROWING EVENTS

1. The throwing area should be surrounded by a protective screen and all spectators and inactive competitors should be kept behind this area.
2. The throwing area should be dry and clean of debris.
3. Participants should never turn their backs to the performance area.
4. No spectators, athletes, or by-standers should be allowed to walk across the field in front of the throwing area.
5. During meets, all participants should follow the instructions of the official who determines when the throwing can safely commence.
6. Participants must warm up before every event.
7. Proper throwing technique should be used to avoid injury.
8. Throwing apparatus should meet regulation standards and be matched to the participants' age, ability, and level of competition.
9. Throwing apparatus should never be thrown directly overhead.
10. Athletes should never attempt to catch a shot, discus, or javelin.

girls use an 8-pound 14-ounce ball, and elementary school athletes use an 8-pound ball.

The circle in which the shot-putter performs is seven feet in diameter and is generally made of concrete.

Practice

Improper technique is the primary cause of injury in this event, so skill instruction should be the emphasis of all practice sessions. Putters must be taught how to gain momentum and release the ball. At first they may try to throw the shot in an overhand fashion rather than push it forward from a position close to the chin. Technique practice should begin without using the shot and then slowly progress through various weight balls until the putter has the experience and confidence to propel the weighted shot-put properly. Novice shot-putters should initially push the ball forward with the hand and then *gradually* progress to the use of the fingertips. They must learn to follow through on the pushing motion after the ball has been propelled forward. Some putters plant their non-dominant foot under the toe bar at the end of their wind-up to stop momentum, gain balance, and avoid fouling. This is an extremely dangerous practice that risks severe leg injuries.

All team members must stay behind a protective screen during shot-put practice. A putter may mistakenly release the ball at any point in his or her wind-up, thereby endangering anyone standing at any point around the circle. Shot-putters should also be prohibited from practicing their event at home. This seriously endangers siblings and neighbors.

Injuries

Most injuries sustained while shot-putting are due to error in technique. Wrist sprain (page 259) will occur if athletes attempt to push forward with their fingertips too early in the season. Hip strain (page 268) happens when athletes give final push to the ball improperly. Muscle inflammation in the forearm will occur if there is a slight imbalance at the time of the final push.

Conditioning

Shot-putting requires body mass, strength, and speed. In addition to the following, conditioning regimes for these athletes generally include sprinting activities (see page 180) to build speed and leg strength, and fingertip pushups to build wrist strength.

Although shot-putters rely on the quick anaerobic energy stored in fast-twitch muscle fibers, they still should engage in warm-ups that focus on the muscles of the shoulders, upper extremities, and lower legs. They should also condition the following body parts:

flexibility (page 67): legs, shoulders, back, hip.

agility (page 71): drills will help develop speed and coordination.

strength (page 72): legs, shoulders, back, hip.

Discus

The discus throw is a twist and whip event. It requires speed, coordination, balance, and strength. It is probably the most difficult track and field event an athlete can attempt to master.

Equipment

Standard smooth-soled shoes are usually used for this event. Some discus throwers remove the spikes (especially from the left shoe) to allow for easier pivoting.

The discus is made of rubber or wood with metal on the outside of the ring. On the high school level the discus used in boys' competitions is of a different weight and diameter than the one used by the girls: the boys' is 3 pounds 9 ounces, with an 8½-inch diameter; the girls' is 2 pounds 3.274 ounces, with a 7 1/16 to 7 3/16-inch diameter. Small spurs which develop in the metallic surface of the discus should be filled immediately to avoid hand injuries.

The discus thrower must gain momentum and throw the discus within a ring that is 8-feet 2½-inches in diameter and is generally made of concrete.

Practice

The discus throw is a well-rehearsed activity. It takes literally thousands of turns to become proficient in this skill. Throwers must learn proper technique. Make sure your athlete has no doubt how to grip, swing, and release properly. Discus throwers must also learn to follow through on the body movement of their throw because sudden deceleration can cause knee ligament injuries.

All team members not involved in the discus throw must be kept away from the area or behind a protective screen. Novice throwers should practice with rubber discs strapped to their hands to allow them to develop a sense of skill and balance while reducing risk of injury to themselves and others.

Injuries

The most frequent injuries sustained in the discus throw are blistering (page 243) or laceration (page 274) of the fingers. Technique practice is important because wrist sprain (page 259) can be caused by an incorrect release movement. Also, the following injuries can occur if the discus is thrown while the athlete is unbalanced: knee injury (page 253), ankle sprain (page 259), shoulder strain (page 268), or shoulder sprain (page 259).

Conditioning

The conditioning requirements of the discus thrower are the same as those for the shot-putter.

Javelin

The javelin throw requires speed, coordination, timing, and strength. The athlete uses an overhead throw and explosive energy to propel the spear forward the greatest distance possible.

Equipment

Because javelin throwers need to run at full speed before throwing the spear, they wear sprinters' shoes or spikes.

The javelin is a lightweight metal spear. The boys' javelin is longer and thicker than the girls', and the placement of the grip determines its distance rating.

Practice

Learning to use speed and strength while maintaining balance takes thousands of practice throws. The goal of running at full speed and throwing the javelin without loss of momentum begins in small steps:

- Throwers need first to learn how to hold the javelin.
- Then they should learn the proper placement of the body and feet to gain muscular support and balance. This is usually done by walking through the motions and then practicing them with a slow jog.
- To gain control and accuracy, the athlete may first practice throwing (without running) into a target area 15 feet away.
- Gradually the skills of running and throwing can be combined as the target area is slowly extended.

Injuries

The most common injury occurring among javelin throwers is the medial epicondylitis at the elbow (page 258). This happens when the arm is not properly warmed up or is not correctly bent enough to put force behind the throw.

Other injuries common to javelin throwers include: fingertip lacerations (page 274), shoulder impingement injuries (page 252), scapular strain (page 268) caused by imbalance at the time of the throw, muscle tear (page 265) caused by sporadic motion in the throw, back and triceps strain (page 268) due to improper warm-up. Anterior cruciate ligament sprain (page 257), which occurs when the athlete attempts to decelerate momentum while turning inward on a planted and slightly bent knee, is also a risk for javelin throwers.

Conditioning

The javelin thrower should use the training workout of the sprinter (page 180) to enhance his or her speed, and should also condition the body in the following ways:

flexibility (page 67): shoulders, back, arm.

strength (page 72): shoulders, back.

Jumping Events

Long Jump

The long jump is an event in which the athlete attempts to combine maximum speed with maximum height to jump the greatest distance. To do this he or she needs speed, spring, coordination, and explosive quick energy.

Equipment

Long jumpers wear track running shoes or sprinter's spikes.

The landing pit is generally filled with builder's sand. This must be turned daily to keep it soft. It should also be raked periodically to smooth over ridges or uneven mounds of sand. (The rake should then be stored away from the pit with the teeth facing down.) The takeoff board should not be wet, loose, uneven, or excessively worn.

Practice

Long jumpers need ample practice on all three phases of this event:

1. The Approach: The athlete must develop speed and learn to pace the acceleration. Reaching maximal stride too soon or too late will cause a strain injury.
2. The Takeoff: The athlete should hit the takeoff board with feet together, heels first, and then go through a standard heel, ball, toe motion. As the center of gravity moves forward, clenched hands should move forward and upward to maintain balance. Early in the season the jumper should avoid repetitive hard jumping. Some jumpers attempt a walking motion while in the air; others tuck in their knees. Your athlete should choose the method that best suits his or her natural motion.
3. The Landing: The jumper must land on both feet with knees partially bent. This position will absorb the impact of the landing and prevent the jumper from falling backwards.

Injuries

Jumpers risk injury if they are insufficiently conditioned or use improper technique. Muscle strain (page 268) can be caused by the sprinter's run on cold muscles. Knee and ankle ligament injury (page 257) may result from improper takeoff or landing.

Conditioning

The long jumper needs the same body conditioning as a sprinter (page 180). He or she also needs abdominal strength (page 72), and should stretch the muscles of the hips, knees, and calf muscles (page 67).

High Jump

The high jump is a ballistic event in which the body is the propelled object. The jumper approaches the high-jump bar with full running strides, then springs up, and rolls over the bar. This athlete needs the speed of a sprinter, the power spring of a hurdler, as well as exceptional balance and coordination.

Equipment

High jumpers may wear shoes that are specially designed for this event, or they may wear standard running shoes with good traction that will keep them from slipping when they plant their foot just before the jump.

The landing pit may be filled with sand, wood shavings, foam rubber mats, or air-filled mats. The approach and take-off area must be dry and well maintained.

Practice

Jumpers must learn and practice each skill of the high jump. These skills include the approach, the planting, the jump, the crossbar clearance, and the landing. To prevent injury to the spinal column, the jumper should learn to land with both arms making initial contact with the mat. This will soften the impact on the back. Participants in this event should be given time to practice the skills of jumping over a very low or even imaginary bar. All jumpers should also be taught the various methods of jumping. They should practice each one and choose the one most suitable to their natural movements. A few popular methods include: the scissor kick, the straddle, and the Fosbury flop.

Injuries

The most common injury sustained by high jumpers is called

"jumper's knee." This rupture of the patellar tendon is caused by the abrupt break from forward motion to vertical lift.

Hamstring and lower back strain (page 268) are caused by saddle jumping with tight muscles. Abdominal strains (page 268) are caused by the twisting motion used in the saddle, western, and belly rolls.

Cervical fractures (page 275) occur when the jumper lands on his or her back (especially when using the Fosbury flop method). Ankle fractures (page 235) happen when the jumper lands off balance.

Conditioning

High jumpers need to condition the body parts stressed by the initial sprinting action of their jump (page 172). In addition, they need the following kinds of training:

flexibility (page 67): hamstrings, quadriceps, lower back.

strength (page 72): hamstrings, quadriceps, knees, abdominal area.

Pole Vault

The pole vault is practiced by male high school athletes only. It is a jumping event that requires speed, upper body strength, coordination, and balance.

Equipment

The size and composition of vaulting poles vary. The length chosen is a matter of individual preference (and availability). Most beginners find it easier to handle a shorter pole, while advanced participants find longer ones (up to an allowable 18 feet) better for height and distance. Fiberglass poles bend and give a catapult-like action to the jump. Older metal poles are stiffer and more difficult to work with, but are often still used in elementary and high school competitions.

The landing pit should be well maintained to ensure safe

landings. The pit should not be covered with fragmented pieces of foam rubber. It should be cushioned with foam rubber mats. The cover of these mats should be routinely checked for tears and holes to avoid water saturation that would decrease their resiliency and shock-absorbent capacity. Also, they should be stored in a standing position in a clean dry place.

All pole vaulters should wear an athletic supporter with a protective cup to protect the genitalia.

Practice

Pole vaulters are sprinters. Their daily practice sessions should include the sprinter's workout described on page 180 as well as the following.

Proper technique for vaulting with a metal pole is quite different than the technique used with a fiberglass one. Make sure your child's coach knows the difference. Regardless of which pole is used, the event is a highly skilled one, so novice vaulters should have at least five to six weeks of practice prior to actual competition. All vaulters must practice how to pace their approach run, how to develop proper stride length, how to plant their pole, how to cross over the bar safely, and how to land. Participants must also learn how to decelerate slowly in order to plant the pole tip effectively, because an abrupt deceleration often causes injury. If the pole misses the mark, athletes must learn how to let the pole slide through the hands rather than risk injury by proceeding with improper execution of the jump.

Injuries

The majority of injuries incurred in this event are caused by improper technique and lack of experience in handling the pole. If athletes attempt to decelerate rapidly they risk suffering anterior cruciate ligament disruption (page 257) in the knee. Improper landing can cause fracture (page 235), strain (page 268) or sprains (page 259) of the lower extremities. If the pole misses the plant site, sudden jarring may lead to shoulder dislocation (page 234) or sprain (page 259). And faulty technique with the fiberglass poles can cause abdominal or hip muscle strain (page 268), cervical sprain (page 259), vertebral and/or skull fracture (page 235), or spinal cord injury (page 275).

Conditioning

Pole vaulters should follow the sprinter's training program listed on page 180. In addition, they should condition the following body parts:

flexibility (page 67): lower back, hips, and abdominal area.
strength (page 72): lower back, hips, and abdominal area.

Considering the high number of participants in track and field events each year, these sports cause few fatalities and have a relatively low rate of injury. Also, because they offer such a variety of events that call on a wide range of athletic abilities, participants have a unique opportunity to find an area of individual competency and enjoyment.

13

■ ■ ■ ■ ■

Wrestling

Wrestling is a nationally popular contact sport that on the high school level alone averages 300,000 to 400,000 participants each year.[1] Unlike some sports that are dominated by certain body-type athletes, wrestling allows for weight-matched participation by athletes of all sizes. But because wrestling ranks third behind only football and basketball in rate of injury occurrence, you need to know what kinds of equipment, practice sessions, and conditioning programs can reduce the risk of injury for your young athlete.

Equipment

Floor Mat

The floor mat should be adequately cushioned to minimize the impact of falls and takedowns. Older mats lose their resiliency and should therefore be replaced. The wrestling mat must be cleaned and disinfected daily to prevent skin infections. When in use, it should also be placed in an area away from other equipment obstacles.

Knee Pads

Knee pads are optional (but recommended) pieces of equipment that are used to reduce the incidence of mat burns (page 273) and bursitis (page 241) of the knee.

Head Gear

Wrestlers are required to wear protective head gear during competitions. You should make sure, however, that your young athletes also wear head gear at practice sessions. These "helmets" are worn to protect the wrestlers' ears from direct blows, friction injuries, and the development of cauliflower ear.

Mouth Guards

A mouth guard or molded wax should be used by any wrestler wearing dental braces. This will prevent lacerations inside the mouth.

Shoes

Although streetwear sneakers are worn by many young wrestlers, specially designed wrestling shoes give the athlete better foot grip on the mat. This not only improves their ability to win, it reduces the risk of injuries that are caused by falls and mat friction.

Practice

When you watch a wrestling practice, look to see if the session emphasizes safety procedures and use of proper technique. The wrestling room should be large enough to allow each wrestling partner ample room to practice without collision with other wrestlers. It has been established that 50 square feet per participant is the minimum space needed to conduct safe practice sessions.[2] Look to see if each practice session begins with warm-ups that emphasize stretching. This will reduce the athletes' risk of suffering twisting and leverage injuries.

A part of the practice session should be dedicated to skill

instruction. Wrestlers must know how to execute and respond to takedowns, sitouts, and standups safely; they should learn how to protect their shoulders from falling impact, and how to stay mentally prepared for each move. They should learn why some holds are illegal and understand the injuries that can occur if they try to struggle out of such holds. A twisting hammerlock can dislocate a shoulder, a full nelson can result in a broken neck, and a twisting toehold can seriously injure the knee. Although in competition these holds will be broken by a referee, young wrestlers need to know what they are and how to handle them.

Because wrestling skills are learned in developmental stages, beginning wrestlers should practice separately from experienced teammates. In this way they can learn the basics without being hurt or intimidated by their lack of ability. For this same reason you should encourage your young wrestlers to attend all practices; there should be no gaps in their training when they go to the mat in a competitive situation.

Because wrestling involves intimate body contact, personal and team hygiene is extremely important. Although it may not be common practice, your athletes should shower before and after every practice and competition and practice uniforms must be cleaned every day. Also, wrestlers with infectious skin problems such as impetigo or herpes simplex (cold sores or fever blisters) should be excluded from practice and competition until proper treatment is initiated and the infection is no longer contagious. Make sure that the mats are washed and disinfected after every practice and competition.

Injuries

The risk of injury is always present in the sport of wrestling. The vast majority of these injuries, however, do not cause permanent damage, nor are they life-threatening. The severity and frequency of those that do occur can be greatly reduced with knowledgeable coaching, skill development, practice, and prompt attention to complaints of pain.

Most wrestling injuries are caused in one of four ways:
1. *Direct blow* injuries can occur when a wrestler makes forceful direct contact with an opponent. They account for a relatively small percentage of all wrestling injuries. Direct blows most often happen when wrestling partners bang heads when they move quickly in the same direction. This may result in a concussion, facial laceration (page 274), broken nose (page 247), or ear hematoma (page 247). If a blow to the ear is left untreated or if the ear is subjected to repeated injury, "cauliflower ear" may result.
2. *Friction injuries* are frequent and often disabling problems for wrestlers. As exposed skin comes into contact with the mat or opponent, mat burns and abrasions (page 273) can occur. These skin problems can easily become infected if the mat is dirty or contaminated and/or if the break in the skin is not promptly treated.
3. Wrestlers often suffer injury in *falls*. Many wrestlers find that during a takedown they can not protect themselves as they forcibly hit the mat. Fractures (page 235), dislocations (page 234), contusions (page 274), sprains (page 259) and concussions (page 246) are the types of injuries that may result from these falls.
4. *Twisting and leverage injuries* can cause wrestlers to suffer sprains (page 259), torn ligaments (page 257), and dislocations (page 234). These injuries occur when excessive pressure is applied to the joints in takedowns or in wrestling moves on the mat. The knee and ankle are the most vulnerable joints because of the twisting involved in takedowns. Hands and fingers are also often injured when the athletes reach and grab to apply or break a hold.

Although the vast majority of wrestling injuries are not life-threatening, wrestling is next to football in causing the highest number of neck and spinal cord injuries. These can lead to fractures, dislocations, or even partial paralysis or quadriplegia. The most common manner of injury results from a compression of the neck while it is slightly bent. For this reason it is especially important that wrestlers learn proper technique and emphasize neck flexibility and strengthening in their conditioning regime.

See page 92 for a list of medical conditions that could prohibit participation in wrestling.

Conditioning

The wrestler most prone to injury is the one who is inexperienced, out of condition, or tired. The goal of injury prevention in this sport, therefore, is to learn proper technique, use a conditioning program that protects vulnerable muscles and tendons, and keep the body strong with proper diet and rest. Unfortunately, because wrestling is a weight-matched sport it has a reputation for promoting quick weight-loss diets that allow athletes to "make weight" just before competitions. As explained in detail in Chapter Five, this practice is a very dangerous one that you and your child's coach should prohibit.

Wrestling is a sport that demands tremendous agility, strength, and muscular endurance. The following exercise regime will give you a sampling of the conditioning program necessary for safe participation:

flexibility (page 67): all-over body flexibility is essential in the sport of wrestling.

agility: (page 71)

muscular endurance (page 72):

strength (page 72): all leg muscles, knees, ankles, neck, and hands.

Wrestling is one of the few sports which relies on individual rather than team effort. Wrestlers can't slide by on the talents of their teammates, nor can they hide in the outfield. Each participant must be motivated to learn and practice the techniques, strategies, and conditioning exercises necessary for competitive participation in this sport. The information in this chapter will help you encourage your young wrestler to do the things that will keep him from injury and make him a winner.

14

■■■■■

Other Sports: Ice Hockey, Lacrosse, Skiing, Swimming, Volleyball

Ice Hockey

Ice hockey is a strenuous, aggressive, and sometimes dangerous sport. To reduce the risk of injury, all participants must wear protective equipment. Young players are required to wear helmets to prevent head injuries which can happen when they crash onto the ice, into the boards, or into each other. This protective head gear should have a face mask of molded bars or a clear shield like those on motorcycle helmets. Ice hockey competitors must also have padded gloves (and should add thumb guards), knee, elbow, shoulder, and hip pads, as well as chest and athletic cup protectors and mouth guards. You should make sure that each piece of equipment is of high quality, fits properly, and is worn correctly. Female players should also wear breast and groin protectors.

205

Like football players, hockey players are liable to every kind of injury mentioned in this book. Bone, muscle, ligament, and tendon injuries often occur from sudden traumatic events. The most common of these include bursitis (page 241) of the elbow, which happens when players break their fall with their elbows; finger and thumb dislocations (page 234); tibial fractures (page 235); ligament tears (page 257) in the knee; and fractures and dislocations of the collarbone and shoulder blade, which can happen as a result of a crash into the boards, a direct blow from a hockey stick or when players collide (a check). Overuse and stress injuries are less common in this sport, but athletes can develop rotator cuff tendonitis (page 281) from the repetitive use of the arm and shoulder movement involved in shooting the puck. This condition is aggravated by practices in which the players hit 50 to 100 consecutive shots.

It is interesting to note that various studies have found that most ice hockey injuries occur in the second half of the game,[1] that forwards are injured more often than defensive players, that 50 to 70 percent of the eye and face injuries result from improper stick use, and that 15 to 25 percent result from fighting or other aggressive acts that are unrelated to actual play.[2]

Because ice hockey requires quick cuts, sudden turns, and sharp moves, your child will need to stay in top physical shape to avoid injury. All practices and games should begin with thorough warm-ups (page 44) that emphasize flexibility exercises (page 67) for the legs, hips, shoulders, and rotator cuff. Because hockey players need quick bursts of energy, they should condition for speed (page 72) to develop their fast-twitch muscle fibers (page 52) and anaerobic abilities (page 52). These athletes should also train for cardiovascular functioning (page 72) and overall body strength (page 72), with emphasis on the leg muscles. Ice hockey coaches generally agree that this is one sport in which the emphasis on conditioning should focus on home exercises. Ice time for practice and play is too expensive to "waste" on body conditioning; therefore the parents of these young players should oversee an off-ice fitness program that will ensure strong and flexible bodies on the ice.

Lacrosse

Lacrosse is a contact sport in which the participants control and move a solid ball that is slightly smaller than a baseball (but just as hard) with a triangular net attached to a stick. They attempt to score a goal by passing the ball past the edges of the goal line. Despite the aggressive nature of this sport, its speed, its stick, and the hard ball it employs, relative to other contact sports there are few serious injuries incurred in lacrosse.

Male players reduce the risk of injury by wearing protective equipment. They are required to wear helmets with face masks and padded gloves. Make sure that your young athlete has a face mask with a vertical bar that prevents the ball from entering and that he uses the chin pad and secures it on both sides. The padded gloves that protect the players' hands from lacerations and contusions (page 274) become essentially worthless when the players cut out the palm side for a better grip. If your son wants his palms free, buy him gloves with pre-cut holes; these will not allow the fingers to become exposed and therefore open to injury. In addition, the goalie must wear a chest protector and a throat protector that is attached to the lower end of the mask. Optional equipment includes arm and shoulder pads. These are recommended to protect players from illegal stick checks.

Female lacrosse players do not wear protective equipment, except for the goalie, who wears a helmet, face mask, padded gloves, chest protector, and leg guards. Because field players are unprotected, the rules for girls' games are stricter than those for boys' and the play is generally less aggressive. It is probable that as girls' lacrosse continues its gains in popularity and includes more bodily contact, the United States Women's Lacrosse Association will introduce protective equipment for its players.

The National Collegiate Athletic Association (NCAA) sponsored a study of lacrosse injuries.[3] The study found an overall injury rate of 52.2 percent. The body part most frequently injured was the shoulder, followed by the knee, ankle, clavicle, and upper leg. More than 70 percent of the injuries were contusions (page 274), sprains (page 259), and strains (page 268). Fractures (page 235) accounted for about 9 percent of the injuries and concussions about 2 percent. Since the lacrosse player wears no protective equipment on the lower extremities, it is not surprising that the majority of the injuries occurred below the waist. Hand and Finger injuries also occurred quite frequently; the researchers who compiled these statistics believed this might happen because the hands and fingers are considered an extension of the stick and therefore are in a vulnerable position, but also because of the custom of cutting open the palm side of the protective gloves.

Surprisingly, the majority of lacrosse injuries are caused by non-contact activities. These occur, for example, when players make a quick turn or sudden cut while running. This fact emphasizes the need for body conditioning before and during the lacrosse season. All players should warm up before each practice and game with flexibility exercises (page 67) that stretch the shoulders, hamstrings, and all other leg muscles. They can also improve their game and reduce the risk in injury by conditioning for speed (page 71) and cardiovascular endurance (page 72). Strength training should place emphasis on the chest, shoulder, and hand muscles (page 72).

Skiing (Alpine)

Alpine skiing is an exhilarating recreational and competitive sport in which participants race down snow-covered hills and mountains at high rates of speed. The degree of enjoyment and safety possible in this sport depends on three factors: the experience of the skier, the ski equipment, and the environment.

Because most novice skiers are young, it is not surprising that the majority of ski injuries are sustained by skiers under the age of sixteen. There are other, not so obvious, factors in this statistic, however, that you can monitor to reduce the odds of injury for your young skier. Many youngsters are injured in ski-related accidents because they use adult ski equipment that is not suitable for their smaller size and lighter weight. Children also often use second-hand, safety outdated, and worn equipment. In addition they are prone to ignore necessary equipment-maintenance procedures and to show off in front of their peers.

These dangerous factors can be eliminated or minimized with competent ski instruction. Frequent and intense instruction at the very beginning of the ski experience is advisable. In addition to skill instruction, lessons should include information on safe ski habits and etiquette, body conditioning, and equipment selection and maintenance.

Young skiers should learn that equipment-related injuries can be prevented by selecting equipment that is of high quality and proper fit, and by following an ongoing maintenance program. The ski bindings in particular must be installed and adjusted properly by a *trained* salesperson or instructor, and they must be kept in optimal condition. Before each use, bindings should be cleaned, lubricated, and tested for ease of release. They should also be covered and protected from corrosion when stored on car roof racks. And, ideally they should be inspected by an expert at least once a year.[4] The ski boot must perfectly fit the skier's foot to prevent ankle sprains (page 259) that are common in skiers who wear loose fitting boots or who don't buckle their boots tightly. Also, the boot should be well padded along the top edge to prevent boot top fractures (page 235). Additional safety equipment that you should encourage your young skier to use includes antifriction devices that attach to the ski between the heel and the toe; these can significantly reduce the incidence of tibial fractures (page 235). Ski straps which prevent the ski from disengaging and spearing the skier after a fall are also recommended to prevent body, hand, and facial lacerations (page 274). The very wise young skier will wear a crash helmet on particularly difficult slopes.

The environment is the third injury-related factor that you must consider when planning for the safety of your young skier. Extreme cold, high winds, poor visability, and icy or bare patches are elements that substantially increase the likelihood of injury. Under these conditions novice skiers should stay off the slopes and all other skiers should exercise extreme caution. When choosing or evaluating ski slopes, look for signs of a continuous maintenance program that keeps the slopes well-groomed. Also, look for evidence of alert and ever-present ski patrols who enforce strict slope discipline and who suspend the skiing privileges of those who ski recklessly or who are under the influence of drugs or alcohol.

Approximately 87 percent of ski injuries are caused by falls.[5] The frequency and severity of these injuries are determined by the three factors discussed above. Most commonly the lower extremities bear the brunt of injuries, with knee ligament problems (page 257) and tibial and boot top fractures (page 235) heading the list. (Ski boots that fit higher up on the leg reduce the risk of boot top fractures, but they increase the incidence of knee injuries.) Injuries to the upper body occur less frequently, but they do happen. Facial lacerations (page 274), thumb ligament injuries (page 222), shoulder contusions (page 274), and clavicular fractures (page 235) are the most common. (Since the introduction of ski poles with flexible grips rather than straps that wrap around the hand and thumb, the incidence of serious thumb and shoulder injuries has decreased.)

Tragically, serious and even fatal accidents can happen on the ski slopes. These accidents are most commonly caused by collisions with fixed objects such as trees, rocks, and chairlift towers. Collisions at high speeds can cause skiers to sustain head and spinal cord injuries as well as internal hemorrhages from lacerations of the spleen or liver. In the vast majority of such cases, the collisions are due to mistakes made by skiers who travel at speeds too fast for their skill level. Before your young athletes take to the slopes, insist that they understand the importance of gradual and progressive skill development.

Safe skiing also requires overall body conditioning. Injuries are more common in skiers who are out of shape and in those who are fatigued and who therefore do not use proper technique. Flexibility, balance, quick reflexes, and above all strength and endurance of the lower extremities are all vital to competent navigation on the slopes. You can help your young skiers keep their bodies conditioned for skiing by encouraging them to follow the conditioning recommendations in Chapter Three.

Note: A newcomer to the ski slopes is the snow board. The management of most ski locations require proof of training and an agility test before they allow anyone to take these boards on the slopes. Whether required or not, make sure that a certified instructor (not a friend "instructor") teaches your child how to safely use this new piece of ski equipment before he or she is permitted to use it.

Swimming

Swimming is both a recreational and competitive sport. It enjoys a reputation as a well-balanced form of exercise that increases muscular strength and tone and contributes to the rehabilitation of a variety of injuries. Although as a competitive sport it requires exceptional skill and dedication, with knowledge of proper stroke execution, early detection of overuse injuries, and proper conditioning, swimming can also be an exceptionally safe sport.

Because swimming is a non-contact sport, swimmers need protective equipment only as a personal need arises. If, for example, swimmers find their eyes burn or become blood shot in chlorinated water, they should wear goggles. Or, if swimmers tend to retain fluid in the outer ear canal (a condition referred to as "swimmer's ear") or have a history of ear problems, they should wear ear plugs. Swimmers with long hair should wear swim caps to keep the hair out of their eyes and mouth. (Caps will also improve speed and help protect hair from chlorine damage.) If your child swims outdoors, be sure he or she wears a sunscreen for protection from the sun's ultraviolet rays.

Despite the fact that swimming is a non-contact sport, injuries do occur. Concussions (page 246), lacerations and contusions (page 274) can occur if a swimmer swims into a wall, or float, or another swimmer. Muscle cramps (page 264) and sore muscles (page 267) are common in unconditioned swimmers. Most swimming injuries of the competitive level, however, are caused by overuse stress on the body's muscles, tendons, and ligaments. The area of stress is determined by the stroke most frequently practiced. The freestyle, butterfly, and back crawl strokes can bring on the pain of "swimmer's shoulder," which is caused by bursitis (page 241), shoulder impingement (page 252), or an actual tear (page 265) of the rotator muscle group. If your swimmer complains of excessive pain around the shoulder or of an occasional "dead" arm feeling, a shoulder instability may exist and should be examined by a physician. The whip kick of the breast and elementary back strokes can aggravate the ligaments of the knee, causing chronic knee pain. Early diagnosis, modification of the leg kick, and a flexibility and strengthening conditioning program will usually reduce or eliminate the pain and allow the athlete to continue swimming the stroke.

Because the majority of swimming injuries result from overuse, conditioning emphasis should focus on general body flexibility and strengthening exercises. Competitive swimmers often use hand paddles or tie their legs to tubes or floats as they swim to build upper body strength. Hand paddles add more resistance to the pull, and a tube or float restricts the leg motion, causing the arms to work harder. Also, because most swimming events call upon the swimmers' fast-twitch muscle fibers (page 52) and anaerobic (page 51) energy supply, competitors should condition for speed (page 71).

Although swimming stands out as an exceptionally safe sport, it does have its tragic side. It is not completely uncommon for good to excellent swimmers (most often males) to drown. Most of these fatal accidents happen to swimmers who are competing with others to see how far or for how long they can swim under water. To prevent this kind of tragedy, explain to your young athlete that without warning extended breath-holding can decrease the partial pressure of oxygen to a point at which the brain can no longer function. When that happens the swimmer loses consciousness and the muscles that control the breath-hold relax. As the unconscious swimmer resumes breathing, he or she takes water into the lungs and if not quickly removed from the water will drown. Keep swimming safe by discouraging all underwater games and exercises that push your children beyond their breath-holding capabilities.

Volleyball

Volleyball has rapidly grown from its place as a recreational beach-party activity to a popular and strenuous sport for males and females. If your young athlete takes up this game you'll find that the safety factors are easily monitored. Although the action of a volleyball game doesn't require body contact, it is classified as a "limited contact" sport because sometimes two or more players will run into each other as they reach for the ball. Players have also been known to crash into the surrounding equipment or walls. These collisions can be avoided and the severity of injury reduced through proper instruction of team play and by padding the net standards, cables, walls, and official's stand.

The only form of protective equipment worn by volleyball players is knee-pads. These are necessary to protect the knees from floor burns and abrasions (page 273). Because volleyball players often fall or slide to their knees to reach a ball, make sure that your young player wears these protective pads and plays on a clean, well-swept floor (to reduce the risk of infecting floor burns and abrasions). Volleyball players should wear a well-cushioned court shoe that gives their arch full support. They should not wear traction sneakers or running shoes because these tend to cause short stops that do not allow participants to slide.

Sprained ankles and fingers (page 259) constitute the majority of injuries in volleyball. Ankles are easily injured when a player lands off-balance after incorrectly executing a spiking or blocking jump. Players who improperly set the ball risk hurting their fingers. Instruction of proper technique during practices will reduce the risk of incurring these injuries. Serious volleyball players who practice and play for a number of years may develop wrist, shoulder, or knee pain caused by an overuse injury. The constant stress on the muscle units of these body parts during repetitive serving and returning drills can cause the athlete to develop an overuse or impingement syndrome (page 252) and can lead to pain in athletes who exhibit even minor shoulder instability. Osgood-Schlatter's disease (page 258) and jumper's knee, which is caused by tendon inflammation (page 281), are very common in 11- and 12-year-old volleyball players.

Although volleyball is a relatively safe sport, the risk of injury can be further reduced with proper conditioning. Volleyball practice and games should begin with warm-ups that emphasize flexibility exercises (page 67) for the shoulders, upper arms, hamstrings, Achilles tendon, and hips. To strengthen leg muscles and improve vertical leap, players should practice the wall jump (page 50). They should also strengthen their shoulders, chest, legs, hips, back, wrists, ankles, knees, and toes. (See strengthening exercises on page 72.) Because volleyball requires players to make quick, sudden moves, players should also condition for speed (page 71) to improve the function of their fast-twitch muscle fibers (page 52) and their anaerobic energy system (page 51).

Part III
Care of Sports
Injuries

15
■ ■ ■ ■ ■

The Young Athlete's Body

Twelve-year-old Jeff Barker loves to play baseball. He's been breaking in his new pitcher's glove since Christmas; he's been throwing snowballs at trees all winter to practice his aim, and now it's finally spring and he's ready to play.

Mr. Barker has taken his son to the field for some pre-practice warm-up. "Come on, Jeff!" he yells. "Keep those pitches coming. You've got to throw hard to practice your control." Jeff's dad and coach both enjoy the boy's enthusiasm; they know they can push him to be the best he can be without a word of complaint. Mr. Barker knows, for example, that Jeff is probably hot and thirsty, but he also knows Jeff won't interrupt their workout to ask for water. "Hey," he figures, "if an old man like me can stand the heat without a water break, I'm sure Jeff is doing fine."

"Lookin' good, Jeff," chimes in the coach. "Now let's see you sprint around these bases. I'll time you. Ready? Go!"

Jeff takes off like a horse free from the starting gate, but as he rounds third, he falls to the ground in pain. As Jeff grabs his thigh and squirms in the dirt, his coach knows he's just lost his star player for opening day. Jeff's dad rushes to his side, wondering how a young kid in such good shape could pull a muscle just by running around the bases.

Many parents and coaches like Jeff's have the best of intentions and would never purposely push their young athletes beyond their capabilities, but because they don't recognize the many ways in which the body of a growing child is different from an adult's, they are often the cause of sports-related injuries.

This chapter will give you an overview of these differences so that you'll better understand the importance of body conditioning, proper sports technique, and safety equipment in the prevention of injuries.

Bones and Cartilage

There is no doubt that physical activity stimulates healthy bone growth in young people. There is concern, however, that intense physical training can interfere with normal bone growth and development. After much debate and clinical study, it is now generally agreed that the immature musculoskeletal system is vulnerable to unique patterns of injury because of the anatomy of the growing bones.

The epiphysis and the apophysis are part of the growth centers found in children's bones. Each has a specific job to do and each is especially vulnerable to injury throughout the body's growing period. A part of the epiphysis called the physis is the growth center that is found at the end of a bone and is responsible for longitudinal growth. Because the ends of a child's bones are made of these cartilage growth plates, rather than being all bone, as in adults, they are more susceptible to injury and are the "weak link in the chain" when an injury occurs around the joint. The epiphysis can become completely separated from the bone; it can also be fractured or crushed.

The vast majority of growth-plate injuries can be treated

effectively and will heal. But sometimes the injury can alter or stop the growth at the epiphysis, which can result in a discrepancy in the length of the involved bone. A partial growth-plate injury can cause an angulatory deformity leading to a decrease in function. Any tenderness just above or below a joint should be evaluated professionally to rule out an epiphysis injury. If a bone injury is not obvious but the pain persists, the athlete should then be re-checked because it is not uncommon for a growth-plate injury to appear negative on an initial X-ray, and to later become obvious when healing begins and new bone is deposited close to the area of injury to support the damage.

The apophysis is found at the point where muscle or tendon attaches to bone. It does not contribute to growth, but it helps the muscles and tendons keep up with bone growth. Apophyses are most often injured by repetitive stress on the growing joint. Problems like Little League elbow (page 262), Osgood-Schlatter's disease of the knee (page 258), and Sever's disease of the heel (page 238) are often attributable to an apophysis injury or inflammation. These injuries are extremely common during periods of rapid growth in the skeletally immature athlete. Sometimes called overuse injuries, these kinds of problems can develop when athletes train too hard too soon. Jeff Barker's dad was trying to help him gain control of his fast ball by encouraging him to throw as hard and as often as he could, but without proper warm-up and muscular conditioning, and an understanding of overuse stress on the elbow's growth center, this practice is doing Jeff more harm than good. An X-ray of an apophyseal injury will reveal a widening or stretching at the site of muscle attachment.

The degree of bone rigidity of the immature skeletal system also affects the kind of bone injuries young athletes sustain. All elements of the skeletal system are formed as cartilage in the embryo. The maturation of cartilage to hard bone (a process called ossification) occurs slowly from about the seventh week after conception to early adulthood. Because children still have a high percentage of cartilage in their bones (while ossified mature bones have a higher concentration of ash), the bones are more flexible than an adult's. This makes a child's bones more susceptible to buckle fractures (page 00) that do not disturb the entire integrity of the bone. It also makes it less likely that they will suffer a compound or open fracture in which there is a complete break in the bone. Associated with the flexibility of children's bones is an injury unique to growing individuals called plastic deformation of the bone, in which the bone bends or deforms but does not break. This requires professional medical attention because these injuries are less likely to straighten themselves as will the angular shape of fractures.

Epiphysis and apophysis growth centers will cease to exist and bones will complete ossification when youths reach maturity: about age 16 in girls and 18 in boys. Until that time the immature skeletal system will react to trauma with injuries that differ in kind from those more commonly seen in adults.

Ligaments

A ligament is a tough band of fibrous connective tissue that joins the ends of bones and stabilizes the joint. Although injuries to these ligaments do occur quite readily in adults, they are rare in children and adolescents. The ligaments of young people are better able to withstand trauma because they seem to be stronger than growth plates, and so it is the growth plate that will most often sustain an injury to the joint.

When a young athlete complains of joint pain, a physician will need to determine if the ligament, growth plate, or bone is involved. Low-impact injuries, like those incurred coming down off balance after jumping to shoot a basketball or spike a volleyball, tend to stretch or tear the ligament from its point of attachment to the bone, especially around the knee and ankle. High-impact injuries, such as those that may occur when a gymnast falls from the parallel bars or an ice-hockey player crashes into the sideboards, tend to apply pressure to the bone itself at the point of ligament attachment and will more likely result in either a growth-plate injury or a torn ligament rather than a bone fracture. Of course, if the force of pressure is great enough, a combination of low- and high-velocity injuries can happen and may result in an injured growth plate along with a torn or stretched ligament. Because joint instability is, as you can see, a complex occurrence, an athlete experiencing joint pain needs professional medical attention to determine the exact point and kind of injury.

Muscles

The muscles of male and female prepubescent athletes are certainly not as strong as those of adults. This seems like an obvious fact, yet in the course of a sports season it would not be unusual to hear a parent or coach insist, "You can throw harder than that!" or "Come on, put some umph in your bat. That ball barely made it to the infield." Very often, young players can not "do better than that" because their muscles simply are not yet strong enough.

As athletes reach puberty, their full strength capabilities will begin to emerge. Male players will begin to produce the male hormone testosterone, which will enable them to build greater muscle mass and strength. Female athletes, however, will never build muscle mass (see page 227 for a full discussion of female muscle strength), but they can build muscle strength through a persistent program of strength training. The average untrained female teenager, however, will not be as strong as her male counterparts. Unless parents or coaches have their girls involved in an intense regime of strength building, it's foolish for them to insist, "If the boys can do it—so can you!" After the age of approximately 12, boys and girls do not exhibit the same degree of muscle mass and strength. This fact should always be taken into consideration when setting sports-related goals and expectations.

In the growth period from prepuberty to adolescence, all children go through growth spurts in which the muscles, bones, and tendons experience rapid growth. Unfortunately for young athletes, this growth is often disproportionate. If a bone grows faster than its muscles and tendons, for example, the joint will lose its flexibility. Athletes who were previously quite limber may suddenly find themselves suffering from strained or pulled muscles. That's why Jeff Barker pulled his hamstring running around the bases before practice started. The year before, he could do that without stretching his muscles first; this year he can't. As explained in Chapter Three, pre-activity stretching is not absolutely necessary for youth league players whose muscles are generally quite flexible. It is a good habit for them to develop, however, because stretching warm-ups are essential for growing junior high and high school athletes.

Thermal Regulation

Studies have repeatedly found that young people are less able than adults to regulate their body temperatures. This results primarily from three physiological facts: children generate more metabolic heat per unit body size than do adults;[1] children demonstrate reduced sweat rates;[2] and children don't initiate sweating until they reach a higher core temperature than an adult.[3] Adults too often assume that because kids are in better general physical health than they, the young athlete should be able to withstand the stress of heat better. This is not so. Fluid replacement in the heat is especially critical for young athletes, who medical researchers know have insufficient thermal regulation. This is especially so in the compromised athlete who already has a fever or a sweat-related disorder such as cystic fibrosis.

Maturation Rate

In all reports of children's sports injuries it is found that injury rate is directly related to increase in age. As a player's age increases, so does his or her risk of injury. Preadolescent players (both boys and girls) follow a relatively consistent and stable pattern of development; therefore, athletes of similar age are generally equally matched in physical size. This enables boys and girls to compete against each other and it allows sports play to remain relatively safe. It's also true that participants at this level of play do not have the speed, mass, or strength to cause significant injury. When preadolescent athletes fall or collide, the forces on their musculoskeletal system are usually not strong enough to cause critical damage. Equal size and low-level impact keep the incidence of serious trauma in preadolescent athletes extremely low.

After about age 12, however, an athlete's chances of incurring significant injury climbs dramatically. This is due, in part, to the fact that players of the same age will exhibit great variations in size and strength. The changing levels of hormones which begin at the onset of puberty cause considerable and often rapid changes in body proportion, muscle mass, and fat distribution. Safe sports competition is most directly affected by these changes because the age at which an individual matures varies from person to person. Some who have not yet started their process of rapid maturation and growth will be on the same team with others their age who have fully completed their physical development. That's why it is not uncommon to see 98 pounds of baby fat and peach fuzz competing against 200 pounds of muscle and mustache.

Expecting teens at early, average, and late periods of maturation to compete equally on teams created on the basis of chronological age is unreasonable. Without full consideration of size and weight (especially in contact sports), participants are deprived of fair competition and are at increased risk for failure and injury.

These uneven matches are also a primary cause of sports burnout. Late maturers who sit the bench or are constantly ridiculed for their smaller size and lesser capabilities come to believe that they are incapable of achieving skilled proficiency in sports. What they don't know and most often don't give themselves a chance to find out is that the early maturing athlete who is the star player at age 12 may not be any better than the late maturer at age 18. One study of a Little League World Series found that 46 percent of the players were postpubescent although all were 12-year-olds or younger. These postpubescent boys, who were two years ahead in average height and weight for age, held down the key team positions.[4] But this early advantage does not continue. A twelve year longitudinal study showed that an outstanding athlete in elementary school has only a 1 in 4 chance to become a sports star in high school.[5]

Knowing the effect maturation rate can have on young athletes' attitudes and health, parents and coaches should consider the state of development to channel a child into sports that are most appropriate for the body size and type. A small thin boy, for example, might have a more positive and healthy sports experience if he joins the tennis, swimming, or soccer team rather than the football or lacrosse team. If your lightweight child insists on playing a contact sport with more mature competitors, however, you probably shouldn't turn him off sports completely by forbidding participation. If you can't persuade your athlete to try a noncompetitive sport, you might do best to monitor all safety factors, such as equipment, practice sessions, and body conditioning, and then use the experience to help your athlete discover personal abilities and limitations.

Female athletes face additional maturation factors that influence their participation in sports. The following section will discuss what you should know about your daughter's physical development and how it affects her ability to play sports safely.

The Female Athlete

Girls are relative newcomers to the sports arena. In fact, 25 years ago the Amateur Athletic Union prohibited girls under the age of 14 from running races that were longer than a half mile, and no woman ran the Boston Marathon until 1967. It was believed that if a girl ran long distances or trained too intensely when she was young, she would become infertile later. It was also believed that menstruating females should not be physically active, that girls could not tolerate heat exposure, and that they were less interested in and needed lesssports play than boys did. All of these beliefs are not true, but still today myths about girls' athletic capabilities persist. Fueling the confusion, Title IX of the Federal Education Act of 1972 mandated equal athletic facilities and programs for boys *and* girls. This implied to many parents, coaches, and athletic directors that boys and girls were absolutely equal in athletic ability. Because female athletes are not too frail to endure intense competition and yet are not on an equal par with male athletes, it's no wonder that parents often have many questions about their daughter's involvement in sports.

Girls vs. Boys

Before the onset of puberty, boys and girls of approximately the same size are equal in athletic capabilities. Because they have the same proportion of muscle mass and aerobic capacity, girls and boys under the age of 12 can play side by side without a perceptible discrepancy in their performances.

During adolescence, however, hormonal changes cause a widening gap between female and male athletic capabilities. The most obvious difference is in their body composition. The male hormone testosterone increases a boy's muscle mass, while the female hormones progesterone and estrogen increase a girl's proportion of body fat. (The average girl has 27 percent body fat, while a boy has only 12 percent.) Due to their smaller muscle mass, lower body weight, and greater fat percentage, females typically have less strength, local muscle endurance, and power than men.[6] In fact the absolute strength of females in the general population is about two-thirds that of males.

A female's maximum aerobic capacity is also affected by her changing body composition. In preadolescence the difference between a male's and female's highest attainable oxygen uptake rate during exhaustive exercise (the VO_2max) is slight. But by adulthood, males have 15 to 25 percent greater oxygen capacity; this gives them an increased capacity for prolonged exercise. This male/female difference in oxygen capacity occurs for a number of reasons. A girl's VO_2max plateaus between the age of 8 and 14, but a boy's will continue to develop until sometime between age 16 and 19. (The closer adolescents are to puberty, the more likely it is that they have reached their highest level of VO_2max potential.) There is also a difference in the average level of hemoglobin and the resultant ability to transport oxygen to the muscles. Because males have a higher percentage of muscle mass, they have a larger stroke volume and a higher concentration of oxygen in the hemoglobin.

Although females are anatomically and physiologically different than males, studies have demonstrated that through training regimes similar to those recommended for male athletes, they can dramatically improve their aerobic capacity, endurance, and strength.

Training

As explained in Chapter Three, aerobic conditioning can improve the ability of the heart, blood vessels, blood, and lungs to supply oxygen to the muscles. Through cardiovascular endurance training, bodily changes occur that help the muscles convert oxygen to energy. These changes include an increase in the number of blood vessels, improved performance of red blood cells, enhanced lung capacity, and stronger chest muscles, which can deliver more air to the lungs with each breath. Aerobic conditioning enhances the respiratory, circulatory, and muscular systems of female athletes in ways that help them compensate for the lack of natural VO_2max development. Sample cardiovascular endurance conditioning exercises are on page 72.

Female athletes can also improve their weaker state of muscle strength through strength training exercises. They can not, however, increase their muscle size because they do not produce the male hormone testosterone. As discussed in Chapter Five, females can build muscle mass only if they use synthetic forms of testosterone called anabolic steroids. But the dangers of such drug abuse far outweigh the advantages. In addition to the dangerous side effects outlined in Chapter Five, females should be particularly alert to the irreversible effects, which include growth of facial hair, a deepening of the voice, and an enlarging of the clitoris, as well as possible permanent changes in reproductive and liver function. Female athletes need to know that steroids can not close the gap between the muscular strength capabilities of males and females. But your daughters can enhance their athletic performances by practicing strength training exercises such as those listed on page 72.

Gynecological Considerations

The majority of female athletes exhibit no change in their performance abilities during menstruation. Some women claim their performances are enhanced at this time of the month, while others feel they are unable to remain competitive during this time. Therefore, no absolute statement can be made about athletic performance during menstruation. Whether your daughters participate, train, or compete while they are menstruating depends entirely on their personal feelings and desires. They should not be forced to be physically active during this time, nor should they be restrained from activity.

Female athletes often begin their menstrual periods at a later age than non-athletes. In fact, it has been found that for each year of intensive training before puberty, a young girl's first menstrual period will be delayed by an average of five months. Although this is a normal occurrence and not a cause for concern, a physician should be consulted if a girl's menstrual cycle does not begin by age 16, or if a once-normal cycle becomes highly irregular.

Menstrual disorders can be directly related to sports participation. They may be caused by a combination of intense training, lowered body weight, reduced levels of body fat, and competitive stress, which can lower the body's core temperature and influence the function of the ovaries and/or the hormonal release from the body or the brain. A woman may be diagnosed as having oligomenorrhea if she has less than 6 menstrual periods in 12 consecutive months; she is said to have amenorrhea if she has less than 2 menstrual cycles in that same time period. These conditions are especially common in endurance sports like long-distance running. Although it may seem desirable to skip the inconvenience and discomfort of monthly menstruation, oligomenorrhea and amenorrhea are relatively unhealthy states because the cyclical shedding of the uterine wall and unfertilized ovum is a natural process which should be allowed to occur. If your daughter experiences menstrual problems, it is important to determine if the irregularity or lack of menstruation is related to athletic activity. If it is, a change in schedule and training intensity, along with relaxation exercises, may alleviate the problem.

Do not assume, however, that a menstrual disorder stems only from participation in sports. A thorough medical evaluation is needed to rule out other problems that present these same symptoms. Menstrual irregularity or amenorrhea can also result from hormonal problems, diabetes, connective tissue diseases, pituitary tumors, thyroid underactivity, eating disorders such as anorexia nervosa or bulimia (page 00), and of course pregnancy.

Any women who develops oligomenorrhea or amenorrhea after puberty should first be considered pregnant. Because it is quite common for a young women to be fearful about admitting a sexual encounter to her parents, a pregnancy test should automatically be included in the medical evaluation of a menstrual disorder.

A full discussion of sports participation during pregnancy is beyond the scope of this book, but you should know that if a young athlete becomes pregnant, it does not mean she can no longer compete in sports. In a controlled environment, with ongoing medical care, physical activity is beneficial for pregnant women.

Injuries

The female anatomy does not make girls especially vulnerable to injury. In fact, a girls' genitalia is less liable to injury than a boy's because it is protected within the pelvis. Breast injuries are also uncommon in athletics, but some girls may feel more comfortable with additional support and/or protection. If your young female athlete wants additional breast support, help her choose an appropriate bra. Flimsy or soft elastic bras offer only a slight degree of support and so are generally useless as sports wear. Tight compression-type bras also do not give the needed support for protection. The most comfortable and desirable bras are those that are made of cotton, are seamless or have no seams across the nipple, have a wide elastic back to prevent slipping and sliding, and have slight padding and structure for protection. Specially constructed sport bras are available at many sporting supply stores for athletes like fencers and long-distance runners who may want more substantial protection than can be found in "street-wear" bras.

The relative frailty of women in strength and cardiovascular endurance also does not predispose them to injury. This fact was substantiated by studies produced by the military academies in preparation to accept female cadets in 1976. The studies concluded that although there were certainly differences in athletic ability based solely on physiological and anatomic differences between the sexes, gross differences in performance capabilities were primarily the result of lack of physical conditioning.[7] Some early studies of injuries in female athletes reported a higher injury rate for females as compared to males. But later studies that compared injury rates of *conditioned* female athletes found no increase in injury over male athletes.[8] This information makes it apparent that although the type and frequency of girls' sports injuries are similar to those of boys, girls must be especially vigilant in their pre-season and in-season conditioning programs.

Benefits

Females derive numerous benefits from physical activity that go beyond the normal health-promoting factors. Contrary to the myth that sports participation endangers reproductive function, it has been found that female athletes have fewer complications of pregnancy, shorter duration of labor, fewer Cesarean sections, and fewer spontaneous abortions.[9] It has also been documented that exercise favorably increases the amount of calcium and calcium turnover in the body. This physiological change in the body has been shown to delay to a significant degree the onset of post-menopausal osteoporosis. Equally important, young girls who participate in sports often develop a life-long pattern of physical activity that will enhance their overall health and the quality of life in years to come. If your daughter wants to be an athlete, you can and should support her efforts without reservation.

16

■■■■■

Specific Injuries and Ailments

Many sports-related injuries can be prevented with consistent and proper use of safety equipment, practice time, and body conditioning, along with parental guidance and supervision. Intense physical activity will, however, always carry the risk of bodily harm. This chapter gives injury-related information that will help you diagnose, treat, and prevent the minor traumas that constitute nearly 95 percent of youth sporting injuries. It will also discuss common overuse and severe trauma injuries that require professional medical attention. The illustrations in Appendix A may aid in your understanding of some of these injuries.

Bone Injuries

Bone Bruise

A mild blow to the body may cause a skin contusion commonly known as a "black and blue" mark. But when the blow is more violent, the impact and subsequent injury may penetrate to the skeletal structures causing a bone bruise. The severity of this injury depends on its location and the force of the

233

blow. Typical symptoms include temporary paralysis of the affected area caused by pressure and shock to the motor and sensory nerves, as well as a hardening of the area due to an internal hemorrhage including the fibrous tissue covering the bone. The skin surrounding the bruise may become "black and blue."

Treatment

- The immediate treatment is the RICE method as explained on page 284.
- Sports play may be resumed as soon as the athlete has no sensations of tingling or numbness to the area and has regained a full range of motion. If the injury involves a lower extremity, there should be no sign of limping.
- After several days, contrast therapy (page 288) can be used.
- As long as there is no underlying fracture, gentle stretching exercises (page 289) should be performed to prevent scarring of any gliding tissue in the injured area.
- A protective pad or guard should be worn over the area as long as the athlete feels discomfort to protect it from further insult.

Prevention

Bone bruises can be prevented with the use of protective padding. Sometimes these pieces of safety equipment are optional wear; athletes who wear all available padding are better protected from this injury.

Dislocation

A dislocation occurs when a bone becomes displaced from its joint. This most often involves the fingers and shoulder joints and can happen when the bone receives a forceful and sudden jolt from contact with another player, an immovable object (like hockey sideline boards), or the ground after a fall. Symptoms include deformity, swelling, pain, and lack of normal movement.

Treatment

- Do not attempt to push the bone back into place.
- Do not give the athlete anything by mouth because he or she may need a general anesthetic later.
- Have the athlete rest and support the injured area with a pillow.
- Immediately bring the athlete to a physician or emergency room. No one should attempt to self-treat dislocations because they often involve a rupture of the surrounding ligaments and tendons; they may even cause small chips of bone to be torn away from the supporting structures, and quite often are accompanied by a fracture.
- Once dislocated, the affected area may be extremely vulnerable to re-injury. Be sure your athlete emphasizes stretching and strengthening exercises in the sport conditioning program to rehabilitate the injured area.

Prevention

The incidence of dislocated joints can be lessened by teaching athletes the skills necessary to safe participation in their sport and by providing proper safety equipment. Athletes should also condition for joint flexibility and strength; however, you should be aware that weightlifting geared to the development of muscle bulk rather than muscle toning and strength conditioning increases vulnerability to joint dislocation, especially in the area of the shoulder.

Fractures

A fracture is a break of any kind in a bone that is caused by a sudden violent insult. The symptoms include swelling, pain, tenderness, lack of mobility, and sometimes deformity. Don't rule out a fracture if your athlete can move the injured extremity and there is little or no swelling; if pain is persistent (over 24 hours) and severe, a mild fracture may exist. Fractures are divided into categories depending on the type of break:

Simple fracture: A defect in the integrity of the bone exists after a specific trauma, yet the fractured fragments are in anatomic alignment. In a simple fracture the bone is broken in one place and does not protrude through the skin.

Compound or Open fracture: The bone is broken in one or more places and the fracture communicates with the skin. It is associated with a puncture wound or a defect in the muscle tissue covering the fracture. A complete discussion of all open fractures is beyond the scope of this book; these fractures range from small puncture wounds to massive amounts of bone and skin loss, with neurovascular damage.

Comminuted fracture: The bone is broken in many places. These may be open or closed.

Buckle or Torus fracture: A fracture in which the bone continuity is preserved but the bony architecture is broken. This only occurs in skeletally immature bones (most commonly in children under the age of 12). Many of these fractures are buckle-shaped, like the torus base of an architectural column, thus the name "torus."

Avulsion fracture: An avulsion fracture results when a piece of bone is pulled off the whole by its muscular attachment. These fractures are commonly found in the knee (especially in athletes involved in sports that emphasize jumping) and at the point where the hamstring attaches to the pelvis. They are also the cause of mallet finger injuries (see page 280). Gentle and persistent static stretching prior to sports participation can significantly reduce the incidence of avulsion fractures.

Epiphyseal fracture: This fracture involves the growth plate of skeletally immature children. There are six major types of growth-plate fractures; each type is diagnosed depending on its location in relation to the growth plate and its prognosis for uneventful healing. A full discussion of the epiphysis is found in Chapter Fifteen.

Stress fractures: These fractures (sometimes called fatigue fractures) result from chronic fatigue, which is usually caused by overuse. Once frequently seen only in military and professional athletes, stress fractures are now common in children. These fractures can occur in any bone subjected to repetitive activity but most commonly affect the tibial leg bone and are therefore most frequently seen in runners who increase their distances too quickly. The pain can occur over a period of weeks to months and is brought on by activity and relieved by rest.

Treatment

All fractures need professional medical attention as soon as possible. If emergency aid is quickly available, do not move the athlete; keep him or her still and as comfortable as possible.

If you must move the athlete to receive medical attention follow these instructions:

- If it is an open fracture, do not attempt to push the bone back through the skin. Try to control the bleeding by wrapping the fracture site with sterile bandages or gauze.
- Immobilize the affected area by applying a splint. To do this attach a firm object such as a board or rolled up newspaper to each side of the fractured area. Make sure that the splint is long enough to include the joint above and below the fracture. Secure with rags, bandages, belts, or anything that will keep the splints together and the bone immobile. This will keep the child comfortable and prevent further damage until professional medical treatment can be obtained.

Jammed Joints

Jammed joints are usually hyperextension injuries to the joints of the fingers (most commonly the thumb and index finger). The symptoms include pain and swelling around the joint area along with a decrease in the range of motion.

Treatment

- Apply ice to injured area.
- Tape the injured finger to the adjacent finger or splint it until the swelling subsides.
- A player should not return to full sport activity until full range of motion has returned to the injured joint.

Prevention

Players can prevent jammed joints by wearing protective hand equipment when appropriate and by learning proper skill technique.

Sever's Disease

Sever's disease is an inflammation of the apophysis (a portion of the bone's growth plate as explained on page 220) at the insertion site of the Achilles tendon into the heel. This causes a traction-type injury that disrupts circulation, causing degeneration and sometimes fragmentation of the apophysis. Sever's disease usually occurs during periods of rapid growth (around age 10 in boys and age 8 in girls). It is most often found in athletes with lean muscular legs who play sports that emphasize running and jumping. Symptoms include heel pain and pain that occurs during ankle extension (especially when the knee is extended). See illustration #1 in Appendix A.

Treatment

Sever's disease is a self-limiting ailment that will take from 3 to 12 months to heal. The following treatment methods may ease the pain and promote faster healing:

- A soft, padded heel-lift or cup added to the inner sole of the athlete's shoe may relieve the pain and allow him or her to continue sports participation.
- Heel cord stretching and ankle muscle strengthening will speed recovery time.
- Only rarely are anti-inflammatory medications necessary. When they are needed their use must be carefully supervised by a physician.

Prevention

Sever's disease can be prevented by gentle and persistent stretching exercises of the Achilles tendon and heel cord prior to sports participation.

Shin Splints

Shin splints is a term commonly used for medial tibial stress syndrome. This involves micro fatigue fractures of the tibia and causes inflammation of the bone itself and of the periosteum (the bone's thick covering). (See illustration #3 in Appendix A.) It most commonly occurs when athletes dramatically increase the amount of their activity or their distance in running without gradual and progressive conditioning. This fatigues the muscles and puts the stress and strain of activity on the bone, which essentially has lost its protective muscular cuff. The injury is characterized by pain on the middle, inside, or outside of the lower leg. This symptom can occur acutely during pre-season preparation or can be a chronic problem that develops slowly over the course of the sports season. The pain can range from mild, after activity discomfort to significant soreness during exercise, to severe incapacitation.

Treatment

- Apply ice massage (page 286) before and after activity.
- Use heat therapy in the form of analgesic packs (page 286) or whirlpool (page 287) to give pain relief.
- Ease pressure on the leg with supportive taping (page 289).
- Pain on the inside of the leg: strengthen muscles that turn the foot in by walking on the outside of the foot and place supportive arches in both shoes.
- Pain on the outside of the leg: strengthen the muscles by running less until the pain subsides. If pain persists, get an X-ray 10 to 14 days after the symptoms begin.
- Pain in the front: do calf stretches (page 69) and wear a soft-heeled shoe.
- Persistent shin pain should receive professional medical attention because it may be a sign of more serious injury, such as stress fracture or muscle herniation.

Prevention

All athletes should wear well-cushioned sport shoes. They should also gradually stretch the ankle and calf muscles before and after physical activity and plan for progressive pre-season conditioning.

Sinding-Larsen-Johansson Syndrome

Sinding-Larsen-Johansson Syndrome is a fragmentation of the lowermost point of the patella which contributes to inflamation and pain in the region of the kneecap. This can lead to tendonitis (page 281) of the patella tendon. (See illustration #3 in Appendix A). While its cause is unknown, it is usually seen during periods of active growth and peaks in rate of occurrence at approximately 8 to 10 years (especially in males).

Treatment

- The RICE method explained on page 284 will ease the pain and swelling.
- Gentle stretching exercises (page 289) for the quadriceps and knee joint will speed recovery.
- Sometimes a knee immobilizer will be necessary to keep the knee completely still and extended.

Prevention

Because this syndrome is a relatively rare occurrence with unknown environmental causes, preventive strategies are not possible.

Bursitis

There is a fluid-filled sac called the bursa that reduces friction in the area between muscles and bones, muscles and muscles, and muscles and tendons. Constant external trauma or overuse of the muscles or tendons at these junctions can cause an inflammation of the bursa and resulting bursitis. Symptoms include swelling, pain, and some loss of function in a joint. Repeated trauma may lead to calcific deposits and degeneration of the internal lining of the bursa.

Treatment

- Initially treat bursitis with the RICE method explained on page 284.

- Forty-two to 72 hours after injury, the area may be treated with contrast therapy (page 288).
- Therapeutic steroid injections should be avoided.

Prevention

Bursitis is most effectively prevented through joint conditioning for flexibility and strength and also with protective padding on joints that consistently receive forceful blows.

Foot Problems

Athlete's Foot

Athlete's foot (sometimes called ringworm) is a superficial fungus infection. This contagious condition is prevalent among athletes because it thrives on the heat, moisture, and darkness of athletic footwear.

Symptoms include extreme itching on the soles of the feet and between and on top of the toes. Fluid-filled blisters or a rash of small pimples will appear.

Treatment

- Treat the feet with antifungal ointment or spray. Over-the-counter preparations are useful in the early stages of infection. (Advanced or chronic cases may need prescribed medication.) Be sure to apply the fungicide thoroughly, especially between the toes.
- Expose feet to air.
- Wear clean white socks to avoid re-infection; change them daily.
- Keep the feet as dry as possible and dust with medicated talcum powder.
- Continue treatment for two weeks after the condition has visibly cleared.

Prevention

All athletes should wear clean white socks and powder their feet daily; they should not go barefooted or wear shoes without wearing socks. Make sure your children dry their feet thoroughly after bathing (especially between and under the toes). If possible, allow sport shoes to air out for 24 hours between use and always spray with an antiseptic spray before each day's wear.

Blisters

Blisters are an accumulation of fluid under the surface of the skin that is caused by friction or pressure. They are a common affliction in athletics. Blisters are likely the culprit when your child complains of surface foot pain that is especially sensitive to the touch. Continued irritation may result in redness, swelling, and eventually infection.

Treatment

Blisters that are less than one inch in diameter and cause no pain should be left alone. Large and/or painful blisters can be treated in the following manner:

- Clean the affected area thoroughly.
- Apply ice for 5 minutes to provide numbness and pain relief.
- To drain the fluid, puncture the blister in several places along the outer edge with a sterile pin or the tip of scissors. (To sterilize, hold over lighted match or dip in rubbing alcohol.)
- Do NOT remove the roof of the blister.
- Squeeze fluid out of the sides by applying pressure to the top.
- Cover with an antiseptic cream and sterile gauze.
- Repeat the procedure once a day for as long as fluid continues to accumulate.
- Apply petroleum jelly over the area if the athlete must continue active participation.

- If the blister is broken before treatment can be implemented, clean the area, apply an antibacterial cream, and cover with a sterile bandage. Repeat this procedure twice a day until the blistered area is healed.

Prevention

Blisters can be prevented by making sure that the sports shoe has sufficient toe room and does not have rough seams on the inside of the uppers. New shoes should be broken in by walking around in them for several days before attempting to use them in active sports play. Susceptible areas can be protected with a liberal layer of petroleum jelly and an extra layer of material such as socks or gloves or bandages.

Calluses

Calluses are caused when constant friction or pressure increases the thickness of the upper layer of skin. Some callus build-up on the hands and feet can protect athletes from skin tears. Excessive callus development, however, can be painful because it causes the skin to lose its elasticity and cushioning effect and may tear, crack, or become infected.

Foot calluses are usually caused by shoes that are either too narrow or too small. If the shoes fit properly and the athlete is still prone to excessive callus growth, he or she may have foot mechanics problems that may require a special orthotic such as a wedge, doughnut, or arch support.

Treatment

- When callus formation begins, athletes should use an emery callus file after each shower and rub on a small amount of lanolin once or twice a week after practice. This will reduce overdevelopment and help maintain some tissue elasticity.
- Once excessive callus growth has formed, a keratolytic ointment may be helpful, or it may be necessary to see a podiatrist who can safely decrease the callus thickness.

• Do NOT attempt to cut off a callus.

Prevention

Make sure athletic shoes fit properly. Routinely apply petroleum jelly to callus-prone areas and wear protective garb such as two pairs of socks or special gloves as used in batting and gymnastics.

Ingrown Toenails

An ingrown toenail is one that has grown into the soft surrounding skin tissue. It is generally caused by tight shoes and improper toenail clipping. Symptoms include severe inflammation, pain, swelling, and redness of the skin surrounding the toenail, and often infection.

Treatment

• Soak the toe in hot water for approximately 20 minutes two or three times a day.
• When the nail is soft, use sterile tweezers to lift the nail from the soft tissue and insert a piece of cotton under the edge. In an alternative treatment, you can cut a small V shape in the upper edge of the nail. Both methods will encourage the nail to pull away from the tender skin.
• Continue the chosen procedure until the nail grows out and can be properly trimmed straight across.
• If an ingrown toenail becomes infected, it needs professional medical treatment.

Prevention

Make sure shoes fit properly. As athletes outgrow their footwear (as young competitors do quite rapidly), pressure on the toenail can cause it to become ingrown.

Trim toenails correctly: 1) cut straight across, not rounded, so that the edges do not penetrate the skin alongside the nail, and 2) leave the nail long enough so that it clears the underlying tissue, but not so long that it can be irritated by sock or shoe.

Head Injuries

The head injuries listed in this section are those that are relatively minor and can be treated at home. However, any head injury that results in unconsciousness must receive immediate attention by a physician. Also, a violent blow to the head can cause skull fracture, cerebral concussion, or spinal cord injuries; therefore, athletes who show signs of nausea, confusion, or disorientation after such a traumatic event need a professional medical examination to rule out serious and even life-threatening injuries.

Black Eye

A blow to the eye can cause internal bleeding that results in the discoloration of a "black" eye. Black eyes commonly occur in sports when an athlete gets hit with a racquet, ball, or an opponent's knee or elbow. The injury needs prompt treatment and rest, but if vision is not affected it should not keep your athlete out of action.

Treatment

- Use an ice pack for 15 minutes and repeat periodically for 24 to 48 hours.
- See your physician if your athlete experiences vision problems such as blurring or an increased sensitivity to light, or if the pupil and iris of the injured eye are not symmetrical with the uninjured eye.

Prevention

Eye injuries can be prevented by wearing protective eyewear as explained in Chapter Four.

Broken Nose

A "broken" nose is actually a cartilage fracture that can occur from a blow from the side or straight on. Immediately after the assault the lacerated mucous lining will cause profuse hemorrhaging and swelling. Deformity is likely when the nose is struck from the side.

Treatment

Control the bleeding (see Nose Bleed) and then seek medical attention for X-rays and treatment of the fracture.

Prevention

When appropriate to the sport, athletes must always wear their helmets with the face masks during all practice sessions as well as competitions.

Competitors should know the importance of staying mentally alert during sports participation.

Ear Hematoma

A blow to the ear can cause an ear hematoma. After such a trauma, the ear will become extremely tender and the athlete will complain of great pain. The ear will also react with pain to environmental elements, especially the cold. If left untreated or if repeatedly injured, the outer ear may appear elevated, rounded, white, nodular, and firm (resembling a cauliflower, hence the name cauliflower ear).

Treatment

- Ice massage (page 286) will temporarily ease the discomfort.
- Professional medical attention should be sought to rule out damage to the inner or middle ear mechanisms.
- Advanced stages of cauliflower ear may need surgical repair.

Prevention

This injury is most commonly sustained by boxers and wrestlers. These athletes should always wear protective head gear that covers their ears.

Nose Bleed

A nose bleed results from a direct blow to the nose or from overexertion. It may affect one or both nostrils. The inner portion of the nose is lined with very delicate mucous membranes, which are affected by changes in humidity levels; therefore, the nose is especially vulnerable to bleeds in very dry regions that promote nasal tissue frailty. Most often the bleeding is a minor problem that is easily and quickly remedied and the athlete can return to sports participation as soon as the bleeding stops completely.

Treatment

• Have athlete lie down with the head elevated and face turned toward the side of the bleeding. This will confine the blood to one nostril and will prevent the blood from draining back into the sinus cavity. Do not let the athlete place head backwards.
• Put a cold compress over the nose.
• Have the athlete use his or her finger to clamp the bleeding nostril and apply pressure for five minutes.
• Instruct the athlete not to blow the nose for at least 2 hours.

Prevention

Athletes must know how to play their position or sport correctly and should stay mentally alert to avoid facial contact. Athletes who are especially susceptible to nose bleeds can lessen their vulnerability with an air humidifier in heated and air-conditioned rooms. This will prevent the drying of the nasal mucous membranes.

Heat-Related Ailments

The body's thermal regulatory system can readily and rather quickly be compromised during athletic participation in a heated environment. Intense physical activity can rob the body of necessary fluids and sodium, which can result in heat exhaustion, cramps, syncope, or stroke. As explained in Chapter Fifteen, children are especially vulnerable to heat-related ailments because their sweating mechanism is not as efficient as an adult's. Most susceptible are those who are obese or anorexic, or who have a fever, suffer from cystic fibrosis, gastrointestinal infection, or cardiovascular problems.

Heat Exhaustion

Heat exhaustion is a condition that causes a thermal regulatory failure when the body overheats due to loss of body fluids through sweating. This can happen when there is excessive heat in the environment or from overexertion.

There are two kinds of heat exhaustion:

1. Thermal regulatory failure can be caused by water depletion. This results when a person accumulates a negative water balance which can happen in a period of just a few hours.
2. Thermal regulatory failure can also be caused by salt depletion. This results when a person develops a negative sodium balance. It usually takes several days for such an imbalance to become evident. To treat this lack of salt, electrolytes must be replaced and so intravenous fluids may be necessary.

The symptoms of heat exhaustion include pale and clammy skin, headache and dizziness, nausea and thirst, near normal to elevated temperature, slow pulse, fatigue and weakness to the point of exhaustion, excessive sweating (decreased sweating in extreme water depletion), and confusion.

Treatment

- Have the athlete lie down in a cool, shady area.
- Loosen or remove clothing.
- Elevate feet slightly.
- Give cool liquids in small sips.
- Apply cool compresses to forehead.
- Drink extra fluids and eat foods like oranges and bananas that are high in potassium.
- Do not allow the athlete to return to activity until all symptoms are resolved.
- Seek professional help if symptoms last more than one hour or worsen, especially when they include nausea, vomiting, and lightheadedness. This indicates a salt depletion and therefore may need medical attention before the athlete returns to sports play.
- Do not let any athlete take salt tablets or sodium-ladened "sports" drinks. It is dangerous to give sodium and potassium supplements immediately after competition (especially if suffering heat exhaustion) except in regulated manner by a physician through intravenous fluids.

Heat Cramps

Muscle cramps can be brought on by intense and prolonged exercise in a hot environment where excessive sweating causes a negative sodium balance. Symptoms include tightening, cramping, and involuntary spasms of the active muscles.

Treatment

The immediate treatment of muscle cramps due to heat exposure is the same as it is for all muscle cramps (page 261).

Once the cramp has subsided, athletes need to replenish the electrolyte and salt loss before they can return to active play. In mild cases of salt imbalance, this can be accomplished by offering a high sodium diet. Severe salt depletion may require the administration of intravenous fluids under a doctor's supervision. Under no circumstances should an athlete take salt tablets.

Heat Syncope

Heat syncope is a condition in which the peripheral blood vessels dilate causing blood pooling and hypotension. The symptoms include giddiness, fainting, skin pallor, and a high (over 103°) body core (rectal) temperature.

Treatment

• Cease all activity and rest in a shady area.
• Replenish lost fluids with water intake.

Heat Stroke

Heat stroke is an advanced stage of heat syncope that may be fatal. It is a medical emergency brought on by dehydration and hyperthermia which causes a complete thermoregulatory failure. Symptoms include a core (rectal) temperature over 103°, a lack of sweating, signs of neurological defect such as disorientation, seizures, and at times even coma. Heat stroke may develop if an athlete is dehydrated and his or her muscle work raises the body temperature to a dangerous level. This raises the temperature of the blood, thereby raising the temperature of the vital organs, especially the heat-sensitive brain.

Treatment

• Immediate professional medical care.

Prevention of all heat-related ailments

Make sure all athletes have an ample water supply to ensure proper hydration prior to activity. Also, provide adequate replenishment during sports participation. Encourage your child to wear light, loose-fitting clothing in hot weather. Do not allow an athlete who has recently had an illness involving fluid loss from vomiting or diarrhea to overexert.

Athletes should not be allowed to exercise in a heated environment for prolonged periods, and should have an opportunity to acclimatize themselves slowly to a sudden change in temperature.

Impingement Syndrome

Impingement syndrome is a term commonly used to refer to injuries in and around the shoulder, especially in the rotator cuff (a group of muscles which cover the shoulder and control its multidirectional abilities). Manifestations of the syndrome can range from edema and swelling to fibrosis (scarring), followed by tendonitis, bone spurs, and tendon rupture.

It is rare to see a true impingement syndrome in a young athlete. But when it does occur, it usually is seen in those who consistently use an overhead motion like that used in swimming the freestyle or butterfly strokes, in pitching a baseball, and in serving a tennis ball.

Treatment

- Rest and activity modification will ease the discomfort.
- Anti-inflammatory medication may be prescribed and supervised by a physician.
- Gentle stretching and strengthening exercises (page 287) will promote healing.
- Corticosteroid injections should never be given to the skeletally immature athlete.

Prevention

Impingement syndrome can be prevented with persistent conditioning of the shoulders, especially by those athletes who use an overhand motion.

Knee Injuries

The knee is one of the most complex of the body's joints. It consists of two long bones, the femur and the tibia. These bones meet and are held together by a series of ligaments, surrounding capsular structures, and menesci (commonly referred to as menescal cartilage). (See illustration #4 in Appendix A.) Because it has little protective padding and is in a vulnerable position the knee is often the site of sport-related injuries.

Knee injuries are of two kinds: *Traumatic* injuries are caused by a blow to the knee area or by sudden twisting. This kind of injury may result in a simple bruise that will not affect the athlete's performance, or it may involve ligament, cartilage, and/or bone damage that require professional medical attention, extensive treatment procedures, and sometimes a lengthy rehabilitation process. *Overuse* injuries, such as Osgood-Schlatter's disease (see below), develop over a period of time.

Treatment of simple traumatic knee injuries

- Use the RICE method explained on page 284.
- Do not apply heat.
- If swelling or pain persists seek professional medical attention. Unattended knee injuries that involve the ligaments and cartilage can lead to serious and even permanent disability.
- Rehabilitate minor knee injuries with ice massage (page

286) before and after flexibility and strengthening exercises (page 289).

General Prevention Strategies

Knee injuries are best prevented with persistent stretching and strengthening exercises.

The use of knee braces as preventive devices is a controversial issue. Several studies have failed to show a decrease in serious knee injuries when prophylactic knee bracing is applied to the knee during sports participation. As explained in Chapter Eight, the only kind of knee braces that seem to prevent injuries are functional ones that are worn to help stabilize a knee that has already had a previous injury.

Cartilage Injuries

Cartilage Tear (Meniscal Injury):

Several joints of the body possess cartilage called meniscus, but by far the most common meniscal injury occurs in the knee. The knee contains two menisci: the medial meniscus is found on the inner portion of the knee while the lateral maniscus is on the outer. Both are attached to the tibia and provide stability to the knee joint in flexion and extension.

A meniscal injury to the knee is often caused by sudden twisting. If a piece of the meniscus is then torn or flipped over and only partially attached, it will block the normal motion of the knee and may even cause it to lock in place. This injury can also cause the knee to "given in" when an athlete is running. A knee that locks or "gives in" or that has tenderness along the inner or outer joint line should be evaluated for a meniscal injury. See illustration #4 in Appendix A.

Sometimes meniscal injuries go hand in hand with ligament sprains. When the medial collateral ligament (page 254) along the middle portion of the knee is sprained, the tibia and femur tend to separate on the inner side of the knee and apply stress to the area of the medial meniscus. (The lateral meniscus is much more mobile and therefore less commonly injured.)

Treatment

In adults, these cartilage structures are almost completely devoid of a blood supply and therefore cannot heal naturally once injured. But in the growing child the menisci appear to be plumper and do possess a blood supply; this increases the possibility of natural and complete meniscal healing (although at times treatment may need to be supplemented with surgical stabilization). These injuries always need professional medical care.

Prevention

Any athlete who has had multiple knee sprains is at increased risk for a meniscal injury. Therefore, those with this increased susceptibility should talk with their physicians about the use of prophylactic knee padding and braces.

Chondromalacia Patella: Chondromalacia patella is a disturbance in the cartilage under the kneecap (patella) or on the surface of the femur bone. As the cartilage in this area weakens, the friction that occurs as the joint moves increases. Because nerve fibers are located at this junction of the cartilage and underlying bone, a disruption in the mechanics of joint motion can become painful. See illustration #4 in Appendix A.

There are three grades of chondromalacia:

Grade I involves a mere softening of the cartilage without gross defect.

Grade II involves some cracking and pitting of the joint cartilage which increases the amount of painful friction in movement.

Grade III involves destruction of the joint cartilage with

exposure and direct contact of the underlying bone to the joint surface.

Symptoms of this cartilage problem include knee pain while walking, running, squatting, and climbing and descending stairs. There may also be swelling around the kneecap and a grating sensation when flexing and extending the knee.

This condition can be caused by a biomechanical malalignment of a joint. The most common type is a patellofemoral malalignment in which the kneecap does not glide smoothly on the joint surface of the femur because of a muscle imbalance or an anatomic malalignment of the leg centered at the knee. Chondromalacia can also be caused by a direct blow or trauma to the knee that causes excessive compression across the surface of the joint cartilage, injuring its blood supply.

Treatment

- Therapeutic exercises may be prescribed to balance the muscles of the quadriceps.
- In extreme cases surgical intervention may be necessary.

Prevention

When caused by sudden trauma, this cartilage problem can be prevented with protective knee padding.

Chondromalacia caused by biomechanical malalignment can not always be prevented. It is known, however, that the problem is most common in females with femoral anteversion. This is a condition in which the axis of the femur bone is set in such a way that there is an exaggerated amount of inward positioning of the thigh bone, often causing in-toeing. Girls who have this problem can avoid chondromalacia through exercises that strengthen the quadriceps. They can also lessen the likelihood of damaging the cartilage by practicing proper sitting posture. Athletes who W-sit (sit back on the knees and

lower legs) can irritate this condition. Patellofemoral malalignment is also aggravated by squatting and therefore by
playing a sports role (such as a baseball or softball catcher)
that requires this body position.

Ligament Injury

There are two major groups of ligaments in the knee. (See
illustration #4 in Appendix A.) The collateral ligaments are
comprised of the lateral and posterior ligaments; these provide
side-to-side stability and permit motion in the knee. The
cruciate ligaments provide the major portion of the front-to-
back stability of the knee. They are strong, fan-shaped structures which are slightly twisted to allow for stability but also
permit motion. Both anterior and posterior cruciate ligaments
are attached to the femur and the tibia. Their function is to
prevent forward displacement of the tibia on the femur. Posterior cruciate ligaments prevent backward displacement of
these bones and hyperextension of the knee.

All ligaments of the knee are very tight when the knee is
extended straight. The susceptibility of these fibers to injury
will vary as the knee bends through different degrees of
flexion. But disruption of the ligaments at any point of relaxation will lead to abnormal motion and rotation of the knee.
Symptoms of injury include abnormal swelling about the knee
area or a sense of knee instability. Both should be evaluated
by a physician.

Like any other ligament in the body, knee ligaments can
become sprained. This is usually caused by an abnormal motion
of the knee joint that places stress on the ligament(s) designed
specifically to prevent this kind of motion. Although all sports
carry the potential for knee injury, knee sprains are most
commonly seen in athletes who are involved in collision sports
such as football or rugby. A full explanation of sprains can
be found on page 259.

Overuse Injury of the Knee

Osgood-Schlatter's Disease:

Osgood-Schlatter's disease is an overuse injury of the knee that is caused by repeated small tears at the point where the patellar ligament connects to the tibia. (See illustration #3 in Appendix A.) This knee problem is found primarily in teenagers: specifically in girls between the ages of 8 and 13, and in boys between the ages of 10 and 15. It has also been found that boys are three times more likely to suffer this injury than girls. Its symptoms include knee pain when kneeling, running, or climbing.

Osgood-Schlatter's disease is one of several pediatric inflammatory problems that affect the sites of tendon attachment into growing areas of the bone. Collectively these ailments are known as osteochondroses.

Treatment

The treatment of Osgood-Schlatter's disease is divided into three stages:

Stage One: Athletes should temporarily refrain from activities that cause pain or aggravate the knee condition. This should relieve the symptoms in 2 to 3 weeks.

Stage Two: If decreasing activity does not ease the knee pain, then the knee should be encased in a soft cast (a knee immobilizer) in an extended position. This will cut down on the strain caused by pulling of the patella tendon on the tibial tubercle and lessen the amount of inflammed tissue over the knee injury.

Stage Three: If Stages One and Two do not stop the knee pain of Osgood-Schlatter's disease the knee must be immobilized in a cast for four to six weeks.

Prevention

To avoid and/or rehabilitate this knee ailment, athletes should engage in stretching exercises that focus on quadriceps, hamstrings, and Achilles tendon. (See page 67 for sample flexibility exercises.) Ice over the affected area may also relieve pain.

Ligament Injuries

Sprain

A sprain is an injury in which ligaments that connect one joint to another are overstretched or torn. In addition, the surrounding and supporting structures may be injured to some degree, causing blood, lymph, and synovial (joint) fluid to rush into the injured area, resulting in immediate swelling. Severed or bruised nerve ends cause pain.

To diagnose and treat a sprain properly you must first determine the extent and degree of the injury. Sprains are classified as Grades I, II, or III.

Grade I Sprain: A Grade I sprain is a mild sprain caused by a minor amount of stretching of the ligaments. The overall continuity of the ligament is intact and there is no gross instability about the joint. There is mild tenderness to the touch, a minimal loss of function, no abnormal joint motion, and little or no swelling. A Grade I sprain does not usually keep the athlete out of action for more than a few days.

Treatment

Mild sprains should not be ignored, because even minor tearing of the ligament fibers has a tendency to recur if left unattended.
- Immediately after injury use the RICE method explained on page 284.
- Follow this with external support such as tape (page 289).

- Use ice massage (page 286) to relieve pain and encourage healing.

Grade II Sprain: A Grade II sprain is a moderate sprain with a partial tear of the ligament. Symptoms include area tenderness to the touch, a moderate loss of function, and a decrease in motion, with swelling and localized hemorrhage. If left untreated, this injury has a tendency to recur and may result in persistent instability and traumatic arthritis.

Treatment

Same as Grade III sprain below.

Grade III Sprain: A Grade III sprain is a severe sprain in which the ligament is completely torn. Stress X-rays will show an abnormal amount of motion in the joint supported by the injured ligament. There is also tenderness, swelling, and hemorrhage along the course of the ligament. At the time of injury a gap may be felt in the area where the ligament is normally located. The injury may be painless, especially if the ligament is completely disrupted. This lack of pain, however, should not be used as a reason to put off professional medical attention. Waiting several hours before obtaining treatment can cause hemorrhaging and swelling that may complicate an accurate diagnosis. Persistent instability and traumatic arthritis can occur if the sprain is left untreated.

Treatment

- Immediately after injury use the RICE method of treatment (page 284).
- The athlete will then need X-rays to rule out the possibility of a fracture; this may be followed by immobilization and possibly a cast or surgical intervention.

- Rehabilitation will involve stretching and strengthening of the injured area (page 289).

Prevention

To prevent sprains, athletes should condition for joint strength. To prevent ankle sprains, all athletes should wear well-fitting and supportive shoes. (See illustration #1 & 2 in Appendix A)

Muscle Injuries

Charley Horse

A charley horse is a muscle tear which causes bleeding within the calf muscle. The athlete will feel intense pain and the area will become swollen and sensitive to the touch. This injury is caused by a direct blow to the muscle or by muscle fatigue and overuse.

Treatment

- Use ice massage (page 286) three times a day. Do not apply heat.
- Slowly stretch while icing.
- Tape (page 289) above, over, and under the area, leaving no openings for blood to pool and swell.
- When sharp pain subsides, begin progressive stretching (page 289).

Prevention

Keep leg muscles (especially the hamstring and the muscles that make up the Achilles tendon) properly conditioned. Wear protective padding when engaged in contact sports.

Epicondylitis

The epicondyles of the elbow are the prominences which you can feel on both the inner and outer aspect of the joint when it is flexed. The forearm flexor muscles attach to the inner (medial) epicondyle, and its extensor muscles and those that turn up the palm attach to the outer (lateral) epicondyle. (See illustration #6 in Appendix A)

Epicondylitis occurs when an irritation develops at these attachment sites or when the athlete suffers a contusion over one of these areas. This is especially common in growing athletes and is often considered a type of Little League elbow (see below). Symptoms include swelling and pain in the elbow area along with decreased range of motion. The pain may be aggravated by a high-five greeting or even a handshake.

Treatment

Epicondylitis can become chronic if it is not treated properly. Treatment includes:
- initial RICE management (page 284).
- rest for the affected arm.
- possible splinting for immobilization.
- At times, anti-inflammatory medications may be prescribed under strict medical supervision.

Prevention

When appropriate to the sport, protective padding can prevent a contusion to the elbow that could lead to epicondylitis. Also, persistent stretching and strengthening of the lower arm and wrist muscles is especially important for athletes who use an overhand throwing action.

Little League Elbow

The term "Little League elbow" refers to an overuse syndrome commonly found in young athletes, especially baseball pitchers. It is caused by the tremendous stress which the throwing motion puts on the inner arm muscle at the place where it attaches to the elbow. (See illustration #6 in Appendix A) This attachment is not as strong in children as it is in adults and so the muscle can more easily be torn away from the bone. This separation can range in severity from mild tendonitis (page 281) to severe destruction of the joint. This injury should not be ignored, because repetitive stress on the growing area (epiphysis) of the joint can cause the child's bone to form in an abnormal way resulting in permanent impairment. Typical symptoms include pain on both the inside and outside of the elbow and mild swelling. If the problem is ignored, the athlete may develop severe pain and find it difficult to put his or her arm out straight.

Treatment

- Initial treatment in the early stages includes rest and ice massage (page 283). Rehabilitation involves stretching exercises (page 287), a possible change of pitching style, and gradual return to full force throwing.
- X-rays are needed to determine the extent of injury. If the condition is advanced, the athlete may need surgery to remove fragments of bone and cartilage that break off and go into the joint.

Prevention

Little League elbow can be prevented. Proper warm-ups and pitching technique are imperative if a young pitcher is to avoid this injury. Also, pitchers between the ages of 9 and 14 should not pitch more than 6 innings each week and should not be allowed to throw curve or breaking balls. Their practice sessions should emphasize low-speed and easy-throw pitching. Athletes can forestall this injury by resting their arm at the first sign of elbow pain and stiffness.

Muscle Bruise

A forceful blow to a muscle can result in a muscle bruise (contusion). The symptoms, treatment, and prevention of this kind of contusion are the same as a skin contusion described on page 274.

A relatively common complication of a muscle bruise is called myositis ossificans. If the muscle is acutely or repeatedly bruised, a hard lump will form as deposits of calcium collect in the muscle cavity. It may take 2 to 3 months for this muscle hardening to become evident. It is most likely to occur in the thigh muscles of soccer and football players and in the upper arm of football quarterbacks.

Treatment

- Any hardened lump should be evaluated professionally to rule out a tumor growth.
- If there is no repeated insult to the area, the lump caused by myositis ossificans may subside completely in 9 to 12 months.
- If the lump does not subside, it may grow into a calcified area which may need surgical removal.

Prevention

Athletes who receive repeated or especially forceful blows to a particular muscle should cover the area with protective padding.

Muscle Cramps

A muscle cramp or spasm is a sudden and involuntary contraction of the muscle. It is particularly common in the neck, back, hamstrings, and calf muscles, and occurs quite infrequently in the arms. The causes are varied and include a blow to the muscle, insufficient conditioning, poor blood supply to the affected area, or excessive salt loss through perspiration.

Symptoms include sudden tightness and pain in the muscle accompanied by lack of mobility. Usually the muscle is not particularly tender and there is no swelling.

Treatment

- Grasp the cramped muscle and squeeze firmly.
- When the spasm subsides, stretch the involved area through its full range of motion and then massage to help restore circulation.
- For calf, arch, or toe cramps, slowly pull the toes toward the front of the leg to a 90° angle. Hold this position until the cramp disappears.
- If cramping is persistent, local heat application with warm pads is helpful. A warm whirlpool is especially useful because it combines both heat and massage to relax the muscle and increase circulation.

Prevention

Include ample salt and potassium (apples, bananas, and oranges) in the diet; condition to increase flexibility.

Muscle Pull or Tear

A muscle pull will happen when the fibers within the muscle are overstretched and rapidly contracted against resistance. If the resisting force is greater than the muscle strength, the fibers may actually tear or rupture. Although any muscle can be injured in this way, the calf, hamstring, and shoulder muscles are more prone than others. The degree of pain, effect on athletic performance, and appropriate treatment depend on the degree of overstretching involved and so muscle pulls and tears are classified into three types.

1) Mild injuries may develop gradually during exercise without causing a moment of acute stress.

2) Moderate injuries result from sudden strain and the pain will cause the athlete to cease activity.

3) Severe injuries are rare, but when they occur they cause extreme pain and total immobilization.

Treatment

Mild injury:
- Decrease level of activity.
- Apply a mode of heat therapy (page 286) before activity and ice and compression (page 284) afterwards.
- If continued activity increases the pain, stop and rest.
- If relief is not obtained in 7 to 10 days, seek professional help.

Moderate injury:
- Stop activity.
- Apply RICE treatment (page 284); continue this for 15 to 20 minutes, 3 to 4 times a day, for 2 or 3 days.
- After 3 days, switch to heat therapy (page 286) for 20 to 30 minutes, 3 times a day. Follow this by gentle stretching exercises (page 289).

Severe injury:
- Stop activity.
- Seek professional help. Surgical repair may be necessary and this is generally followed by extensive physical therapy for rehabilitation.

Prevention

To prevent muscle pulls and tears, athletes should plan an off-season conditioning program that provides for cross-training of the muscles not ordinarily developed in their sport. This will give them balanced muscle flexibility and strength.

Conditioning will also help prevent muscle injuries. Athletes must warm up properly before activity. They should also be careful not to progress through a conditioning program too rapidly or enter a sports season without pre-season conditioning.

Muscle Soreness

Muscle soreness can vary in intensity from mildly annoying to severely debilitating. It can begin during or immediately after exercise; or it may appear 8 to 48 hours afterward. Immediate soreness is caused by stress-induced ischemia in which the muscles are depleted of oxygen and so pain and spasm ensue. This impairs the muscle's ability to quickly remove metabolic waste products, such as lactic acid and potassium, and these accumulate to cause pain. With rest, blood flow increases and the pain eventually disappears. Delayed soreness may result from tissue tears or irritation, local muscle spasm, or gradual lengthening of the muscle. This delayed-symptom injury requires the more intensive treatment stated below.

Symptoms of muscle soreness include localized pain in the specific muscular area which is tender to the touch and will hurt when stretched or exercised.

Treatment

- Rest the sore muscles, because continued intensive physical activity can cause a more serious injury and delay recovery.
- Apply warm whirlpool (page 287), followed by progressive stretching (page 289) and ice massage (page 286).

Prevention

Athletes can avoid muscle soreness by habitually practicing warm-ups and cool-downs (page 44). They must also base all workouts on the principles of progression and overload (page 41).

"Stomach" Cramps

This pain in the side of the abdomen (sometimes called a "stitch") often occurs while running. The discomfort will increase if the athlete continues the pace. It can be caused by loss of salt and potassium through perspiration, overexertion beyond the level of physical fitness, spasm of the breathing muscles, or it may be the effect of taking blood away from digestion for use in the active muscles.

Treatment

- Stop running as soon as the cramp occurs.
- Apply pressure with the hand directly on the area of pain.
- When the pain is completely relieved, the athlete may return to physical activity.

Prevention

Drink fluids before and during sports participation. Avoid eating 2½ hours before physical activity. Add salt to foods. Limit sweets and increase intake of potassium-rich foods such as bananas, apples, and oranges 12 hours before exertion. It may also be helpful to eat foods high in carbohydrates one day prior to the sports event. Condition to increase aerobic capabilities.

Strain

A muscle strain is similar to a ligament sprain. It is an injury in which the muscle suffers undue stress or tension. It is diagnosed as one of three types, depending on the severity of the symptoms.

First Degree Strain

A mild or slightly pulled muscle that is associated with a low-grade inflammation and some disruption of the muscle-tendon tissue.

Treatment

- Immediately after the injury occurs, use the RICE method of treatment (page 284).
- Follow this with external support such as a splint or tape (page 289).
- Use ice massage (page 286) to relieve pain and encourage healing.

Second Degree Strain

A strain in which there is tearing of the muscle fibers without complete disruption. It is usually caused by a violent contraction or excessive forcible stretch. The symptoms include pain aggravated by movement or by tension placed on the muscle, moderate muscle spasm, swelling, impaired muscle function, and "black and blue" skin discoloration.

Treatment

- Use the RICE method described on page 284.
- Gently and gradually stretch the affected area.
- The athlete should not return to activity until he or she is completely without pain and has full range of motion and strength in the strained muscle.

Third Degree Strain

The most severe type of strain; it will usually cause a prolonged disability. It is an injury in which there is ruptured muscle or tendon, with separation of the muscle from muscle, tendon, or bone. Sometimes the injury may involve a pulling away of the muscle and tendon from their attachment site on the bone. The symptoms include severe pain, spasm, swelling, tenderness, loss of function, "black and blue" skin discoloration, and a palpable muscle defect.

Treatment

• This most severe strain requires aggressive medical intervention that may include surgical repair.

Prevention

Gentle stretching and strengthening exercises of all major muscle groups will condition the body to ward off muscle strains.

Tennis Elbow

Although the pain of tennis elbow is felt in the elbow, the source of the problem is in the wrist muscles. The muscles that flex and extend the palm and those that move the fingers begin at the elbow joint. (See illustration #6 in Appendix A) Through overuse, the microscopic attachment sites of the muscles and tendons at the elbow may become inflamed. If the muscle is forced to continue working, it may actually tear away from the bone. The stress on the muscles is generally caused by improper technique, poor conditioning, or an ill-fitting racquet grip. Symptoms include pain on the outside of the elbow during gripping, especially when hitting backhand shots, or pain on the inner aspect of the elbow when hitting forehand shots.

Treatment

• Rest the injured arm. This will mean a cessation of play until the muscle has time to heal and be rehabilitated. The length of time required to do this depends on how long the athlete has played while in pain, thereby increasing the severity of the injury. For this reason, players should rest the arm as soon as they feel pain; this will reduce the amount of time necessary for healing.
• Ice massage (page 286) 3 times a day, 20 minutes on and

at least 20 minutes off before and after activity to reduce swelling.
• Slowly stretch wrist muscles by moving wrist in all directions.

Prevention

Tennis players can avoid this elbow pain by learning proper swing technique. They should also use a racquet grip sized to fit their hand and they should strengthen wrist muscles by holding a 2- to 4-pound weight while flexing and extending the wrist.

Skin Infections

Herpes Simplex

Herpes simplex is a virus that is caused by a skin and mucous membrane infection. Type 1 herpes is generally found on the lips (commonly called a cold sore or fever blister) or on the side of the face, neck, or shoulders. Type 2 herpes is found in the genital area. Both can, however, be found anywhere on the skin or mucous membrane. This viral infection is extremely contagious and is usually transmitted directly through a lesion. Lesions generally occur 24 hours after an infected athlete feels hypersensitivity and swelling in the area. He or she may feel generally ill with a headache and sore throat and lymph gland swelling. The lesions will rupture in 1 to 3 days and leave a yellow crust. They will clear up within 10 to 14 days.

Treatment

Athletes with herpes need professional medical care. The infection can not be "cured" but certain prescribed courses of treatment can reduce the pain and promote self-healing.

Prevention

Herpes is so highly contagious that it has been known to run through an entire team in a very short time. Athletes involved in body contact sports such as wrestling or basketball should not participate with any athlete suffering these lesions. Infected players should be barred from activity for at least 5 days.

Impetigo

Impetigo is a bacterial infection of the skin. It is characterized by small lesions that form into pustules and then form yellow crustations.

Treatment

- Wash the area several times a day using a medicated cleansing agent and hot water to remove the crustations.
- Dry the area thoroughly.
- Apply an antibiotic cream or prescribed medication.

Prevention

Because impetigo is a highly contagious disease, infected athletes should be isolated from all players until the contagious period has passed. This is especially important in body contact sports, such as wrestling and basketball, where there is skin exposure. All players should avoid sharing gym clothing, uniforms, and towels.

Skin Wounds

The injuries to the skin most commonly incurred in sports participation are abrasions, contusions, lacerations, and punctures. These wounds are usually readily treated and healed and seldom require prolonged absence from sports play. If proper treatment is not immediately given, however, some may become infected and then the athlete faces a longer and more painful recovery. When evaluating the healing progress of skin wounds, look for signs of infection, which include tenderness to the touch, redness, swelling, and possibly fever. These symptoms can occur anywhere from one to seven days after the initial injury. To prevent serious infection, be sure your athlete is currently immunized against tetanus.

Abrasion

An abrasion is an irritation of the surface skin layer caused by friction; the outer layer of skin may be completely rubbed off. This is commonly referred to as a "skinned knee" as well as a *floor* or *mat burn*. When players involved in sports such as tennis, volleyball, or basketball fall and slide on the court, they often come up with floor burn abrasions of the skin. Wrestlers and gymnasts suffer mat burns in the same way. These injuries seldom bleed, but the injured surface will turn red.

Treatment

- Although abrasions are minor wounds, if they become infected this simple irritation can become a serious problem. Therefore, regardless how loudly your athlete protests, cleanse the area with soap and water and dry thoroughly.
- Apply antiseptic ointment.
- Cover with sterile gauze pad.

Prevention

The risk of suffering abrasions is drastically reduced when athletes wear protective skin pads on their knees and elbows.

Contusion (Bruise)

Contusions result when tiny blood vessels in the tissues are broken by a hard blow. Alone, they are simple to treat, heal rather quickly, and do not keep an athlete from participating. If, however, they are complicated by an accompanying fracture or involvement of internal organ, professional medical attention is needed.

Treatment

- Follow the RICE method explained on page 284.
- Heat therapy (page 286) 24 hours after the initial injury may ease the pain.

Prevention

Sport-appropriate protective padding will reduce the risk of contusions.

Laceration

A laceration is a cut in which the skin is torn open and the edges are jagged. This injury will bleed and the surrounding area may swell and become tender to the touch. The severity of the cut determines if the athlete needs professional medical attention.

Treatment

- Apply pressure directly over the wound to stop the bleeding. This is best done with a clean towel.
- If the bleeding stops, the cut should be cleansed with warm soapy water, covered with an antiseptic cream, and bandaged with a sterile gauze pad. The cut should be cleaned and re-bandaged every 8 hours.
- If direct pressure does not stop profuse bleeding within 10

minutes, the athlete may need stitches to close the wound. He or she should seek professional medical attention.

Puncture

A puncture is a wound caused by a sharp piercing of the skin. These injuries most commonly result when an athlete is stepped on by another athlete wearing spiked shoes. The severity of these wounds depends on their location and the depth of penetration.

Treatment

Puncture wounds generally need professional medical treatment because it is difficult to clean out properly the dirt and germs that often become lodged deep beneath the skin. If the wound is not completely cleansed and properly medicated and bandaged it will become infected and cause the athlete unnecessary pain and debilitation.

Spinal Injuries

Spinal cord injury is the sports-related catastrophe most feared by coaches and parents. It has been well publicized that severe neck injuries can cause paraplegic or quadriplegic paralysis in young, formerly healthy and robust athletes. Although this does happen, it is interesting to note that sports-related spinal cord injuries are less common than those caused by motor vehicle accidents (38 percent), falls or jumps (16 percent), and gunshot wounds (13 percent). In fact, only diving represents a significant number (9 percent) of sports-related spinal cord injuries, while American football and trampoline injuries each accounts for approximately only 1 percent, and ice hockey, rugby, and gymnastic activities each accounts for less than 1 percent. Although spinal cord trauma rarely occurs in sports, it does happen. And so, as a parent, you need to know something about this devastating occurrence.

The incidence of major spinal cord injuries increases significantly through childhood, peaking between 15 and 18 years of age. The reason for this peak period is believed to be twofold. First, it is during this age period that the number of youngsters involved in sports is at its highest point. Due to the simple mathematics of participation, teenagers are more susceptible to neck injuries than any other group. Second, the skeletally immature spine of younger athletes is more flexible and therefore more resistant to injury. Unlike younger athletes, however, by age 18 the area most susceptible to cervical flexion lies between the fifth and seventh cervical vertebrae. A flexion injury in this area is the most common cause of major neurological damage, thus making the older athlete more at risk.

While it is unlikely that significant spinal cord injuries will ever be eliminated from sports completely, the majority of the activities that place participants at risk have been identified. With this knowledge in mind, changes in equipment design and requirements, along with safety-conscious rule changes have greatly decreased the incidence of these injuries. Continued research, education, knowledgeable supervisors, and trained coaches will continue to reduce the occurrence of these dreaded accidents.

One word of caution: only qualified and trained medical personnel should remove the helmet from an athlete who has injured his or her head and neck. There are many documented cases in which a helmet or piece of head gear was removed from an athlete, who although in pain showed no obvious neurological problem, which resulted in acute flexion of an unstable spine, causing quadriplegia. If your athlete complains of neck pain, do not allow anyone to touch the head gear until a trained professional arrives.

Burner

A burner is a contusion of the spinal cord which may involve the cervical spine and the group of nerves which join as they exit the spinal cord (the brachial plexus). These nerves supply both motor and sensory function to the neck, shoulders, and upper extremities.

After suffering this kind of injury (which usually occurs after head to head contact), the arm hangs at the side with pain primarily in the shoulder. The athlete may feel a burning (hence the name "burner"), tingling, or numbness, or even loss of function or sensation in the upper extremities which can last from several seconds to 30 minutes. If this ever occurs, and the pain and discomfort last more than several seconds, or if there is a decrease in sensation or obvious weakness, even if temporary, the player should be strictly prohibited from returning to play until evaluated by a physician.

The latest studies and statistics in sports medicine suggest that an athlete who experiences multiple burners should have an MRI (magnetic resonance imaging) evaluation of the cervical spine to rule out spinal cord injuries as well as the possibility of a variation in the diameter of the neck (cervical spine stenosis). Athletes who have a slightly narrower spinal canal in the area of the neck are more susceptible to this injury.

If the weakness persists, it is not uncommon for physicians to recommend evaluation by a neurologist or rehabilitation specialist, who may continue evaluation with an electromyogram (EMG) and a nerve conductive velocity test, which measures the response times of muscles and nerves to stimulation in comparison to the opposite unaffected extremity.

Treatment

All burners need professional medical attention. If an athlete experiences a burner and it is not completely resolved within a minute or two, he or she should not go back into sports activity until evaluated by a physician. If two burners (even if short-lived) occur during a single event, the player should be restricted from play until a full neurological workup is performed.

Athletes who continue to play despite the fact that they have experienced multiple burners and have been advised by their physicians to discontinue contact sports participation may develop permanent weakness in their arms and a strength deficit in their upper extremities.

Prevention

Burners are prevented through proper use of technique in all contact sports. Any athlete who has experienced a burner for 30 to 60 seconds should wear a neck roll to prevent recurrence.

Sunburn

Sunburn is caused by overexposure to the sun. Its symptoms include a reddening of the skin that becomes tender to the touch.

By the age of 20, most individuals have received 80 percent of their lifetime exposure to the sun. The cumulative result of sun exposure during the early years is primarily responsible for the later damaging effects of the sun's ultraviolet rays, which include premature aging of the skin, wrinkling, and skin cancer. If your athlete is engaged in an outdoor sporting activity, make sure that he or she is well protected from these destructive rays. This is especially important for youngsters with lightly pigmented skin. The areas most likely to be damaged by the sun's rays are the face, top of the ears, and the back of the hands.

Treatment

• Treat the burned skin with cool compresses.

- Reduce the pain with aspirin or acetaminophen. The pain will peak 6 to 48 hours after exposure.
- Apply over-the-counter sunburn cream or spray to ease the pain and promote healing.
- Apply lubricating creams only after 24 hours, as they may retain heat.
- If the athlete experiences dizziness, fever, blisters, impaired vision, or extreme pain, seek professional medical help.

Prevention

Make sure your outdoor athletes wear sunscreens with a protective factor of at least 15. Rub this into the vulnerable areas mentioned above at least one hour before exposure to allow time for skin absorption. Make sure they wear this lotion whenever they're outside. The damaging ultraviolet rays will penetrate clouds and haze. If possible, have your athlete avoid practice sessions between the hours of 10 A.M. and 2 P.M.

Also, if you have the option, choose uniforms and practice clothes that are of a tightly woven material rather than a porous loose weave.

Synovitis

Synovitis is an inflammation of the synovial membrane, which secretes a fluid to lubricate the joints. This may be caused by an injury to the joint or by systemic causes such as rheumatoid arthritis, lupus, hemophilia, and certain tumors. Synovitis can also result from a variety of other causes such as arthritis, trauma, and/or an immunological response to a viral illness. The symptoms of this inflammatory disease include pain and swelling in the affected joint and increased skin temperature around the joint area. There is also a decreased range of motion in the joint. Many times (especially in the knee) the joint can not be fully extended or flexed because the joint capsule is distended with fluid.

Treatment

- This joint problem is best treated with rest and curtailment of any physical activity that aggravates the swelling and pain.
- Anti-inflammatory medication may be administered under strict medical supervision.

Tendon Injuries

The tendon is a tough cord of dense white fibrous connective tissue that joins a muscle with some other part of the muscular unit and transmits the forces exerted by the muscle. Most often, chronic tendon injuries are caused by overuse.

Mallet Finger

A mallet finger is caused by an injury to the last (distal) joint at the end of a finger. If the tip of the finger is hit forcefully, the extensor tendon may pull off the bone, causing the last joint to drop down. The athlete will not be able to bring the joint back up and fully extend the finger.

Treatment

- Immediately following the injury, apply the RICE method explained on page 284.
- Once X-rays verify the diagnosis, the finger will be splinted. Although this splint must stay in place for at least 3 months, most athletes can return to play as soon as the swelling and pain have subsided.

Prevention

This injury often happens when a player catches a ball with the fingertips rather than with open hands and palms. Proper technique and protective hand gear may prevent mallet finger from occurring.

Tendonitis

Tendonitis is an inflammation of the tendon either at the point of insertion into the bone or at the junction of the tendon-muscle attachment. This inflammation can be caused by a direct blow or by overuse of a muscle group which has not been conditioned prior to participation in the sporting event. Symptoms include swelling, pain, and tenderness to the touch.

Treatment

• Immediately apply the RICE method explained on page 284.
• Use gradual and gentle stretching as explained on page 289.

Cortisone injections are sometimes used to control or curtail the inflammation of tendonitis. However, these injections should not be administered to young athletes. Although cortisone can dramatically reduce inflammation, it can also degrade normal tissue fibers and weaken the area of the muscle/tendon and bone/tendon junctions. Tendons that have been treated with cortisone have a much higher incidence of rupturing and then require surgical treatment.

Prevention

To avoid tendonitis, it is especially important for athletes undergoing preadolescent growth spurts between the ages of 10 and 12 to perform stretching exercises of all major muscle groups prior to activity.

Sometimes tendonitis can be associated with an accumulation of calcium in the area of injury or inflammation. This condition is referred to as calcific tendonitis and may present as a bone spur.

Tenosynovitis

Tenosynovitis is an inflammation of the tendon and its surrounding sheath. In its acute state there is rapid onset of pain, joint crackling, and swelling. It is the result of a direct blow to a tendon and/or insufficient stretching prior to activity.

Treatment

- To ease the pain and swelling of this condition, athletes must rest the affected musculotendonous unit.
- Initial ice massage (page 286) may be prescribed to decrease pain and swelling.
- Steroid injection should NOT be used to treat tenosynovitis.

Prevention

Athletes can prevent this tendon inflammation by stretching properly and attaining an appropriate degree of flexibility prior to all physical activity.

Tendon Rupture

Tendon ruptures occur when there is a complete tear in the tendon. They can be caused by the injection of steroids into a tendon, by a direct blow to the area, or by a sudden violent flexion or extension of a joint. They are common in brittle diabetics undergoing dialysis. Ruptures can occur in three locations: 1) at the bone-tendon junction, 2) at the tendon's midsection, and 3) at the musculotendonous junction. These ruptures usually present with signs of severe pain with a palpable gap in the area. This pain will last for several minutes until swelling, muscle spasms, and blood fill in the defect and relieve the area of an obvious void.

Treatment

A tendon rupture requires immediate professional medical attention. Athletes with suspected tendon injuries should not be allowed to return to active play until the problem area has been thoroughly evaluated.

Prevention

Tendon ruptures caused by steroid injection can obviously be prevented by discontinuation of the practice. The incidence of tendon ruptures caused by the more common cause, direct blows, can be significantly lessened through the use of protective padding, generalized stretching prior to activity, and strict adherence to proper technique.

17
■ ■ ■ ■ ■

Rehabilitation of Sports Injuries

Rehabilitation is a program of therapeutic treatment that strives to return athletes to their level of pre-injury fitness. Because many young competitors want to return to their sport before they are fully healed, you need to take the responsibility for keeping your partially healed athletes off the playing field. Returning too soon puts them at risk for re-injury and perhaps permanent disability. At the same time you can encourage them to take an active part in their rehabilitation and help restore the disabled function as quickly as possible.

The rehabilitation program will vary according to the injury, its severity, and chosen method of treatment. The following information is presented to explain how and why rehabilitation works. Use it to support and clarify the advice of your doctor and coach/athletic trainer as you guide your injured athlete back into action.

RICE

The initial treatment for most minor injuries such as sprains, strains, contusions, and questionable fractures is found in the acronym RICE:

R = Rest

As soon as an athlete is injured, he or she must stop participation and rest the injured area.

I = Ice

When severe trauma such as spinal cord or head injury has been ruled out, immediately apply ice bags or cold packs over the injured area. Cold causes blood vessels to constrict; this lessens the swelling and inflammation by reducing blood circulation to the area. As the fluid pressure on the nerve endings eases, pain is reduced. Keep the ice in place with an elastic wrap or bandage. Be sure there is something between the ice and the skin to avoid frostbite.

C = Compression

Make sure the ice pack is held firmly against the injured area. This compression will further reduce swelling and inflammation. Initially, an elastic bandage can be wrapped directly over the ice. If there is numbness and pain when the bandage is applied, loosen it a bit.

E = Elevation

For 6 to 8 hours following the injury, the athlete should try to keep the affected area elevated whenever possible. When elevated, gravity will drain fluids away from this area and continue to reduce the swelling and inflammation. The level of elevation does not have to be drastic; to assure correct treatment, raise the involved area just high enough so that an imaginary ball could roll from the injury downward toward the body. For example, if the ankle is hurt, raise it up just high enough so that a ball could roll from the foot to the hip.

Use the RICE treatment initially for 30 to 35 minutes. Then remove the cold compress and apply an elastic wrap for support and compression, and keep the area elevated. Repeat the RICE treatment 3 times a day, 30 minutes on and at least 30 minutes off for 24 to 72 hours (depending on the doctor's recommendation and the degree of pain). Discontinue cold compress at bedtime and sleep with the injured area propped up for continued elevation. Re-apply the elastic wrap in the morning and continue the keep the injured area elevated whenever possible.

Ice Massage (Cryotherapy)

Ice massage is an effective way to continue the cold therapy of the RICE treatment after the initial pain and swelling have subsided.

Freeze a paper cup full of water. Rip away the top portion of the cup to expose a half-inch of ice. Move the ice over the injured area to create a massaging effect for 10 to 15 minutes. Repeat every 2 hours for 5 to 10 minutes.

Cryotherapy can be accomplished by this kind of ice massage or by cold water immersion of the injured area, or with ice packs, chemical cold packs, or flexible gel cold packs. Whatever method you use for applying cold, the physiologic effects will be the same.

Heat (Thermotherapy)

Heat can be used to increase circulation to the injured area, relax muscles, and relieve muscle spasms. It should only be used 48 to 72 hours *after* injury; earlier application will increase the amount of swelling.

Hydrocollator packs (purchased over the counter at drug stores) can be used to apply heat. These silicon packages are heated in water (but not boiled!), wrapped in several layers of towels, and placed on the injured area. Heating pads, as well as hot towels that are wrung out, wrapped around the area, and covered with plastic can also be used.

Heat therapy should be used with low-temperature heat and for no more than 15 minutes, 3 times a day. Excessive temperatures may be temporarily soothing, but will encourage swelling and hypersensitize the nerve endings in the area. In the long run this will delay recovery and return to sports participation.

Hot baths should be used with caution because total immersion in *hot* water can be dangerous. Heat channels blood to the skin and away from other vital organs. When the athlete stands up, the blood to the brain may be momentarily cut off, causing him or her to faint and then drown.

Whirlpool (Hydrotherapy)

After acute pain and swelling of muscular injuries, sprains, strains, fractures, and contusions have subsided (generally 12 to 24 hours), whirlpool treatment can quicken the rehabilitation process by decreasing muscle spasms and by massaging and temporarily increasing blood circulation to the recovering area. This mode of rehab is most effectively applied to athletes whose treatment involved immobilization and to those recovering from injuries that have left them with some muscular stiffness. The goal of whirlpool therapy is to help these players regain a full range of motion and flexibility.

With the growing popularity of in-home whirlpools and jacuzzies, many parents wonder how they can use them as rehabilitation aids. The following guidelines will explain how to use forced water as a mode of treatment, but be sure to check with your physician before attempting self-treatment.

- Use cold water for all new injuries. Cold will help reduce the swelling and pain.
- After 48 to 54 hours, or for old or chronic injuries, use warm water.

- If possible, submerge only the injured area. Full body immersion can result in unconsciousness if the immersion period is too long or the water too hot. Whether submerging a body part or full body, limit your athlete to a maximum of 15 minutes at a temperature of 105°.
- When using the whirlpool after an injury, direct the spray toward the side of the tank; a direct spray can cause additional bleeding. Twelve to 24 hours after first use, the forced water flow can be directly applied to gain massage benefits. Encourage your athlete to stretch the injured area gently or tense the injured muscle during the whirlpool treatment. If pain persists after hydrotherapy, apply ice massage (above) for 15 minutes.
- If you do not have access to a whirlpool, your athlete can gain similar benefits by placing the injured area under a running faucet or shower.

Combined Therapies

A common rehabilitation regime involves using a warm whirlpool treatment, followed by gentle stretching (see below) of the injured area, and finishing with 20 minutes of ice massage.

Contrast therapy alternates cold and heat applications. The pumping action of alternately speeding up and then slowing down circulation helps decrease swelling. This method is helpful when a significant amount of swelling is present and a full range of motion is lacking and so the athlete requires a desensitization of pain as well as a soothing deep heat to encourage joint movement. This method involves placing the injured area in cold water for 1 minute and in hot water for 3 to 5 minutes. Four or five cycles several times daily are most helpful.

Massage

The manipulation of muscles through massage can bring an injured athlete reduced swelling, relaxation, and an increase in range of motion. All of this is of course desirable, but an overzealous or incorrectly applied massage can aggravate an injury and increase the pain and swelling. Massage should never be used on a bruised area and not until several days after the initial occurrence. If you want to try an at-home massage, check with an athletic trainer or your doctor for instructions on how to do it properly.

Tape Support

Taping is used to support injured ligaments and joints. It can also be used to maintain bone and joint alignment. You should know, however, that proper taping is a technical and practiced skill that should not be attempted by an untrained person. Moreover, even in the best of circumstances tape support has been found to be effective for no longer than 10 to 15 minutes during activity.

Therapeutic Support

Therapeutic advances are contributing to more rapid sport-related rehabilitation. Air and gel splints, for example, are often used to support ankle injuries. They provide a stirrup effect, giving medial and lateral support by allowing the ankle to flex up and down, while at the same time preventing the ankle from reproducing the movement which caused the injury. These lightweight supports make it possible to put weight on the foot sooner than usual after an injury. This helps reduce swelling and maintains muscle strength. Because prolonged inactivity weakens muscles, making the already damaged ankle even more vulnerable to re-injury, the movement made possible by these "casts" can reduce healing time for severe sprains from the usual 3 to 6 months to 6 to 8 weeks.

Stretching and Strengthening

Progressive stretching and strengthening are necessary steps in the rehabilitation of muscle weaknesses caused by soreness, cramps, pulls, tears, strains, or contusions. Because healing muscles scar, if they are not stretched they may actually shorten or suffer varying degrees of atrophy. Once a muscle regains its full range of motion, it needs to be strengthened before it can perform at its pre-injury level. As soon as your athlete can perform an isometric contraction of the injured muscle (such as tensing or pushing down on a hard surface) without pain, he or she should begin stretching exercises.

Rehabilitation can also be enhanced if your injured athletes have access to an isokinetic machine such as the Cybex, Kin-Com, or Biodex. They should be instructed to start with high-speed/low-resistance exercises and should repeat these exercises daily for as long as they are not in significant pain. They can then gradually progress to low-speed/high-resistance exercises. Although this will encourage muscle strength, the use of these machines can be dangerous unless supervised by experienced personnel such as certified athletic trainers or registered physical therapists.

If you do not have access to such machines, muscles can be stretched and strengthened by following this rehab program:

1. Begin slow stretching to the onset of pain (do not bounce). Hold at that point while *gently* increasing the stretch over 15 to 20 seconds.
2. When flexibility begins to return to the injured muscle area, add isometric exercises (page 63). Tense the muscle only to the point of pain. Hold for 10 seconds and relax for 10 seconds. Repeat the exercise for 2 to 3 minutes. Do not push through pain. Continue isometrics until athlete has regained full range of motion without pain in the injured muscle.
3. Begin strengthening the muscle with isotonic exercises (page 63). Use weights that are light enough to lift without pain. Lift, moving muscle through its full range of motion in one direction over 5 seconds and then back again over

5 seconds. Rest for 10 seconds. Repeat for 2 to 3 minutes. Do not lift in pain. Gradually and progressively increase load only to a point that produces no pain.

4. Start slowly practicing the skills of the sport in a non-competitive environment. Begin running, throwing, swimming, and so forth. Gradually increase practice moves to half maximum effort and then finally to full effort.

Moderation is the key to successful rehabilitation. "Babying" the injured area can result in atrophy, inflexibility, and delay in healing due to circulatory impairment, but working "through the pain" can also delay recovery by causing further damage to the already compromised body part. Make sure your athlete faithfully follows a gradual program of stretching and strengthening and stops at the onset of pain.

5. Ease back into play. Athletes who return to sports participation before they can go full speed, or while still favoring their injury, are at risk for re-injury or related problems. Before returning your competitor to action make certain that the injured area meets the following criteria:

- pain-free motion
- full range of motion that is equal to the opposite body part
- pre-injury level of strength
- normal coordination of movement (no limping, favoring, and so forth)
- little or no swelling

Chiropractic

While the application of chiropractics in the health maintenance of athletes is distinct from that of orthopedics, it is evident that bone and muscle manipulation is playing an ever-increasing role in adolescent, college, and professional sport programs. This became obvious at the 1990 Superbowl football game between the San Francisco 49s and the Denver Broncos.

Just prior to the game the most valuable player, Joe Montana, was interviewed while he was being conditioned by his chiropractic physician.

The basic philosophy of chiropractics and its role in sports participation and rehabilitation include the maintenance of a well-balanced musculoskeletal system from a biomechanical and strength point of view. Spinal as well as major joint manipulation is often performed both prior to and after competition, as well as during the stages of injury recovery.

The vast majority of sports-related injuries can be readily treated and rehabilitated to bring the athlete back to pre-injury condition. The process in youth athletes, however, needs your supervision. Even simple injuries, if not properly healed, can turn into chronic problems that will interfere with optimal performance for years to come. Also, while following a rehab program, don't let your child neglect the uninjured body parts. All muscles need to be kept in shape so that the athlete is completely ready for action when he or she returns to the playing field.

CHART 17.1
MODES OF REHABILITATION

Therapy	Effect	Indication for Use	Application	Time Intervals	Precautions
RICE	• reduces circulation • eases fluid accumulation on nerve endings	initial treatment for most minor injuries such as sprains, strains, contusions, and questionable fractures	R = rest I = ice C = compression E = elevate	3Xs a day, 30 minutes on, at least 30 minutes off for 24-72 hours	• Do not use until severe trauma like spinal cord or head injury has been ruled out. • Do not put ice directly on skin. • Do not compress area too tightly.
Ice Massage (Cryotherapy)	• reduces circulation • reduces pain and swelling	use after initial pain and swelling have subsided	freeze a paper cup of water massage ice over injured area	initially 10-15 min.; repeat every 2 hours for 5-10 minutes	• Keep ice moving to avoid frostbite or skin burn.
Hydrocollator Packs (Thermotherapy)	• increases circulation • relaxes muscles • relieves muscle spasms	use 48-72 hours after muscle or ligament injury	heat in water (not to boiling); wrap in layers of towels and place on injured area	no more than 15 minutes 3Xs a day	• Never apply immediately after an injury. • Do not use over eyes or genitals. • Do not overheat the skin.
Whirlpool (Hydrotherapy)	• cold: reduces circulation; relieves pain and swelling • warm: increases circulation; relaxes muscles; relieves muscle spasms	cold: use after 12-24 hours to continue reduction of pain warm: use only after acute pain and swelling has subsided (48-54 hours)	if possible, submerge only affected area	maximum of 15 minutes with temperatures no higher than 105°	• Do not direct full force of water on a new injury. • Full body immersion in hot water can cause an athlete to faint.
Contrast Bath	• cold slows circulation; • heat speeds circulation; • pumping effect helps decrease swelling.	use 24-48 hours after injury	put injured area in cold water (40-50°); then in hot water (max. 105°)	1 minute in cold; 3-5 minutes in warm; alternate beginning and ending with cold.	• Watch for increased swelling or pain when in warm water.
Massage	• increases circulation • relaxes muscles • increases range of motion	use 48-72 hours after injury	use a lubricant; move motion toward the heart	5-10 minutes	• Never massage a bruised area. • Do not use immediately after injury. • Should be administered with correct technique.
Tape Support	• supports injured ligaments and joints • maintains bone and joint alignment	use on unstable joint 24-48 hours after injury	must be correctly applied by trained personnel	———	• Recognize limited effectiveness during activity.

18

■■■■■

Sports Participation for Chronically Ill and Handicapped Athletes

All children need exercise because physical activity is vital for healthy growth and development. But if your child suffers from a chronic physical or mental health problem, you may wonder if sports participation should be restricted or encouraged. Consider Eric's case. Eric had suffered from asthma since he was born. His parents were well acquainted with the hospital emergency room, where they would frequently rush him in the dark of the night for a shot of adrenalin when his wheezing and labored breathing could not be controlled with his prescribed medication. Now, at age 7, Eric wants to play organized baseball, but his parents can't agree on whether or not Eric's asthmatic condition should exclude him from sports participation. His mother worries that physical exertion, especially during the hot and humid days of baseball season, might bring on severe asthma attacks. But Eric's father doesn't want Eric to miss out on the fun and comradery of sports play and he also believes that playing baseball may improve Eric's state of health. Eric's mom may be right, but then again his dad may be right—it depends on the level of oxygen concentration in Eric's blood. Only Eric's physician can determine that. This is why questions of sports participation by children like Eric, who have chronic health problems or handicaps, should be dealt with on an individual basis through a medical evaluation that is tailored to the child, the health problem, and the specific sport.

Although no blanket statement can be made as to whether these children should or should not participate in sports, most physicians agree that athletic exercise is especially beneficial for most of these children. Because they often feel isolated from their peers and therefore have a low self-esteem, the American Academy of Pediatrics has noted that children with chronic health problems can use sports to enhance their self-image, provide a sense of accomplishment, develop a sense of competitiveness, and establish social and emotional relationships with their peers.[1] While it's true that children with health problems are sometimes limited in their ability to participate in intensely strenuous activities, and therefore may not excel in highly competitive sport situations, it's also true that when these athletes have their physicians' okay to compete, and when they understand the limitations imposed by the illness or handicap, and when they have a strong desire to join an athletic program, there may be greater risk to physical and mental health in denying them activity than in permitting them to participate.

The physical and mental health problems discussed in this chapter are ones that commonly affect sports participation. The information, advice, and suggestions that follow are based on the latest research and recommendations by the American Academy of Pediatrics and the American Academy of Orthopedic Surgeons. Occasionally, however, there is controversy over sports participation by chronically ill and handicapped children. So be sure to consult your physician before your child engages in sport activities, and don't hesitate to get a second opinion if a physician recommends exclusion from athletic participation.

AIDS (Acquired Immune Deficiency Syndrome)

Some controversy exists over the advisability of allowing young athletes with AIDS to participate in sport programs. Although exercise is an important factor in maintaining optimal health in all children, strenuous physical activity may pose a serious health risk to those infected with the human immunodeficiency virus (HIV—the virus that causes AIDS). Because this virus weakens the immune system, infected athletes who become fatigued, injured, or who simply contract a common illness like the flu or strep throat may find themselves faced with a health crisis. For this reason children with AIDS are encouraged to choose non-strenuous sport activities. (See page 91 for a list of non-strenuous sports.)

Although there is no reason to bar HIV-infected children from sports participation, some coaches and parents worry that the virus may be transmitted to other players. These worries are understandable but unfounded. Innumerable studies have concluded that HIV can not survive in air, or water, or on things people touch; it survives only in the blood, tissues, and in some bodily fluids of infected people. Unlike the chicken pox and the common cold viruses, the AIDS virus spreads only if infected fluids go directly into the blood or body tissues of another person. Even if infected athletes cough, or sneeze, or vomit, or spit, or bleed near other athletes, the teammates or opponents are not in danger of contracting the virus because they have not taken these things directly into their own bodies. This assertion is supported by 8 studies conducted of 500 people who lived with people who had AIDS. The 500 people shared toilets, toothbrushes, dishes, bed linens, and towels with infected individuals. Not one single person got the AIDS virus.

Of course common sense dictates that players should use

caution to avoid coming into direct contact with an infected player's bodily fluids. Even though not a single case of transmission through saliva has been documented, it does contain very small amounts of HIV. Therefore, players should not exchange mouthpieces or drink from common water barrels. It is also prudent for players to refrain from sharing any sweat- or blood-saturated equipment. There is no doubt that AIDS is the most frightening epidemic of our day, but keep in mind that no one has ever become infected by playing sports with an infected athlete.

To find more information about AIDS, you can call the National AIDS Hotline at 1–800–342–AIDS, 24 hours a day, 7 days a week.

Diabetes

Children with controlled diabetes should be allowed to participate in all sports activities. However, because the key to controlling diabetes is in the control of blood sugar levels, insulin-dependent athletes must learn how to schedule their insulin injections and food intake on a timetable that regulates the body's sugar level during physical activity. Contact your physician to establish this timetable before your young athlete begins athletic training. Most often diabetics need to increase their food intake before and after sports participation to prevent hypoglycemia, which can occur if the body can't meet the demand for additional glucose energy during periods of physical exertion. If active involvement exceeds 30 to 40 minutes, these athletes will also need snacks during sports play. Give your young diabetic snacks such as raisins, orange juice, or glucose tablets that can be taken inconspicuously before, during, and after physical activity and yet will not load him or her with the empty sugar calories of a candy bar.

Your physician may also want to adjust the dosage and the site of the insulin injections. Because regular periods of exercise can naturally increase the body's level of glucose, diabetics may require a reduction of insulin dosage on days of sports participation. Diabetic athletes who depend on insulin injections may also need to choose a new injection site that is not likely to sustain trauma during sports play. For example, the forearms and thighs are inappropriate sites for football and soccer players because these areas of the body are often open to collision. Tell your physician what sport and what position your child wants to play and together choose a safe injection site.

Sports participation may actually be considered a desirable component in the treatment of diabetics. While exercise will not improve diabetes itself, it offers benefits that enable the child to attain better overall fitness. As it does for all athletes, exercise improves the level of circulating fat in the body, as well as enhances cardiac and respiratory functioning. In addition, exercise is especially beneficial to overweight diabetics. These children need the physical activity of sports play to expend extra energy, reduce daily caloric intake, and lessen the insulin resistance often associated with obesity.

You can obtain more useful information about diabetes and sports participation from the Diabetes America Association. The local branches are listed in the white pages of the telephone book.

Down's Syndrome

Perhaps the biggest advancement in the last ten years regarding sports participation by children with Down's syndrome has come through a better understanding of potential instability in the area of the cervical spine and its articulation with the skull. The American Academy of Pediatrics recommends that at the age of 5 or 6, children with Down's syndrome should have a screening X-ray of the neck in the neutral position as well as in flexion and extension. The spinal measurements that are made between the head and the cervical spine as well as the elements of the upper cervical spine will indicate if an instability exists.[2]

These X-rays should be evaluated before the child with Down's syndrome is allowed to participate in contact sports. It is generally considered safe to say that if no instability is present on the X-rays, participation in sports may be allowed with minimal or no follow-up as long as the participant remains asymptomatic. If the measurements do note an instability of the spine, sports which involve a potential for trauma to the head and neck should be restricted and the cervical examination should be repeated every two to three years. Restricting contact activities will usually suffice as effective treatment. Occasionally, surgical stabilization will be recommended, however, if continued contact sports participation is desired.

For more information about sports play for children with Down's syndrome call this national helpline number: 1–800–221–4602.

Epilepsy

The nature, severity, and frequency of your child's epileptic seizures are the primary factors to consider when deciding his or her appropriate level of sports participation. Although there is still some debate on this issue, considering the effectiveness of newer anti-convulsive drugs, it is rare that a child with controlled seizures should have to be excluded from participating in *any* sport. In fact, for these children, sports participation may lessen the frequency of seizures because many epileptics have fewer seizures when they are active than when they are sleeping or resting.

However, a child who has daily or even weekly major psychomotor seizures (grand mal) should be encouraged to choose non-contact sports. (See page 91 for a list of non-contact sports.) This recommendation is not made because there is any danger that hitting the head will trigger a seizure, but rather because a sudden fall into unconsciousness during a contact athletic event could result in serious injury.[3]

The Epilepsy Foundation can give you more specific information about epilepsy and sports play. Look in the white pages of the telephone book to locate a branch in your area.

Hernia

There is no evidence to support the theory that sports participation will increase the potential of hernia strangulation or incarceration. Therefore, there is no reason to exclude an athlete from physical activity on any level of sports involvement if he or she develops a hernia. Even athletes involved in strength training can continue but should be careful to tailor the workout so that it does not put undue stress on the groin or abdomen and aggravate the condition. A physician may, in fact, recommend delaying treatment until the end of the sports season so that the athlete will not be sidelined during the surgical recovery period. Limitation of activity should be based solely on the athlete's level of discomfort.

Hypertension

Children with hypertension (high blood pressure) can and should participate in sports programs. Their participation should be carefully supervised, however, and these athletes may need to limit their involvement to certain sports. Blood pressure levels rise continuously from birth to adolescence so it's important that athletes with hypertension remain under a physician's care because the exact upper level of normal blood pressure in children is not known. For practical purposes of comparison, the general guidelines of upper limits are:

130/75 for individuals under 10 years of age
140/85 for individuals 10 to 15 years old
145/90 for individuals 15 to 20 years old.

Children who meet or exceed these limits should undergo a stress test (like the Harvard Stress Test or a cardiovascular stress test on a treadmill) before participating in strenuous sports. (See page 91 for a list of sports classified as "strenuous.") If the results of this test indicate that your child is suffering from extreme hypertension, the physician will most likely exclude your child from sports play until the condition can be treated (probably with medication) and brought under control. If, however, the stress test indicates that your child has mild to moderate hypertension, participation in sports that offer aerobic exercise will be beneficial to his or her condition. Aerobic exercise (such as found in distance running and swimming events, as well as bicycling, basketball, and soccer) has a proven therapeutic effect on factors which contribute to hypertension, such as weight control, blood pressure, and fat-level profiles. The athlete may also find that the blood pressure level lowers as he or she gains increased cardiovascular fitness through exercise.

No athletes with any level of hypertension should engage in intense strength training or weightlifting. These activities are known to cause dramatic elevation of blood pressure and would be especially dangerous to athletes who can not safely endure increased systolic or diastolic pressures. A physician may also exclude from activity athletes who suffer organic hypertension which is caused by conditions such as kidney problems or vascular abnormalities.

Physical and Mental Handicaps

Children who are physically and/or mentally handicapped need and enjoy sports play just as non-handicapped children do. Although it is well known that sports involvement can help these children develop coordination skills and an improved sense of self-esteem and self-confidence, unfortunately it is not uncommon for them to be excluded from participation. This accounts, in part, for the emotional problems, lack of coordination, obesity, and general lack of fitness sometimes found in handicapped youths.

Despite the obstacles often encountered in finding outlets for organized sports participation, parents should make an effort to involve their handicapped children in some kind of group physical activity. And just like parents of non-handicapped athletes, they need to monitor and provide for a program that considers individual age, abilities, level of coordination, and degree of physical fitness and health.

The Committee on Sports Medicine of the American Academy of Pediatrics has found that mentally handicapped youngsters usually find a greater degree of success participating in individual and dual sports rather than in team sports, and in activities that require gross rather than fine motor coordination. Therefore they often especially enjoy swimming, hiking, camping, soccer, tennis, bicycling, folk dancing, and boating.[4] It is also known that whether competing with their peers or playing with neighborhood children, the mentally handicapped can better reap the benefits of sports participation when they interact with those of the same developmental level rather than the same chronological age.

Physically handicapped athletes also can and should join competitive teams in a variety of sports. Sport teams for amputees, for example, include skiing, swimming, and running. Those confined to wheelchairs can also play in organized wheelchair leagues in sports such as basketball and cycling. (See Appendix B for a list of sports for handicapped athletes.) The Special Olympics program has also shown us that physically and mentally handicapped athletes can compete successfully against their peers. It's also true that many can and should join non-handicapped children in non-competitive physical activities.

You can obtain information about planning recreational programs for handicapped youngsters by writing to the Information Research Utilization Center for Physical Education and Recreation for the Handicapped, c/o American Alliance for Health, Physical Education and Recreation, 1900 Association Drive, Reston, Virginia 22091.

For more information about the Special Olympics, write to: Special Olympics, 1350 New York Ave., N.W., Suite 500 Washington, DC 20005.

Respiratory Ailments

Asthma

Athletes with asthma should have an exercise stress test to determine their level of oxygen saturation before they participate in any strenuous sport activity. (See page 91 for a list of sports classified as "strenuous.") The result of this test will dictate what degree of activity an athlete may engage in without risking an asthma attack. Although intense physical activity may trigger an asthma attack, studies have consistently found that progressive exercise training in children with asthma results in an increased capacity for exercise and demonstrates a gradual improvement in symptoms and a decrease in the frequency of wheezing. Short intense workouts that are followed by rest periods are more likely than sustained exercise periods to offer these benefits.

The phenomenon of exercise-induced asthma (EIA) appears to be the cause of the majority of asthma cases in young athletes. Although its exact cause is not clear, researchers who have studied the effects of air quality on athletes believe that ozone pollution contributes to EIA. Pollution is known to irritate the lining of the lungs and so, they reason, as exercise increases the rate at which one brings air in and out of the lungs, the lungs become more intensely irritated. Studies have found that inhalation of even so-called "unpolluted" air during workouts causes exercise-induced asthma in 20 to 50 percent of today's athletes. Obviously, those exercising in ozone-polluted areas run an even greater risk of developing this ailment. Given this information, it is apparent that the environment in which an asthmatic athlete is exercising should be given careful consideration when choosing a sport. A dry, pollution-free environment is more desirable than a warm, humid, and/or smog-filled space.

Asthmatic athletes can usually control their condition during periods of physical activity in a number of ways. They can learn specific ventilatory muscle endurance training exercises that will increase their tolerance for exercise. Symptomatic relief may also be found by practicing exercises in which the asthmatic breathes through the nose rather than the mouth. Asthmatic athletes should also have prescribed inhalants on hand during athletic activity to prevent asthma attacks from escalating.

Under a doctor's supervision, asthmatic children and adolescents can benefit from exercise in a number of ways. Although sports participation can not improve the level of pulmonary function, it can definitely improve endurance capabilities, fitness level, and VO_2max. When the asthma is not exercise-induced, researchers have also found that physical activity can improve school attendance and even lessen the severity of a child's emotional response to the asthmatic attack.[5]

Your local chapter of the American Lung Association can give you more information about asthma and sports participation.

Cystic Fibrosis

Like asthmatics, children with cystic fibrosis should undergo stress testing prior to sports participation. Under appropriate medical supervision, children with this lung disease generally can and should enjoy moderate levels of physical activity. Although to date there are no scientific studies to document the benefits of exercise for youths with cystic fibrosis, there are reports that exercise programs which encourage deep breathing can enhance the production of cough and sputum and give benefits similar to vigorous pulmonary physiotherapy.[6]

Extra caution should be used, however, if the child with cystic fibrosis attempts strenuous activity in warm weather. Cystic fibrosis is characterized by excessive sweating of perspiration that contains abnormally high amounts of sodium and chloride. This hypohydration and salt deficit may bring on heat exhaustion or even heat stroke. These athletes must be especially careful to drink fluids before, during, and after sport play.

For more sports specific information, contact the Cystic Fibrosis Foundation in your area.

Sickle Cell Anemia

There is a distinction between having the sickle cell trait and actually having sickle cell anemia, which does affect a child's ability to participate in sports. No evidence to date supports the belief that athletes with an asymptomatic sickle cell trait are more susceptible to injury or sudden death than any other athlete. Therefore children who have been diagnosed as possessing the sickle cell trait, but have no symptoms of the disease, should not be excluded from any level of sports participation.

Children *with* symptomatic sickle cell anemia, however, need to be closely monitored during periods of physical activity and should completely avoid contact sports and strenuous activities which may place them in a sickle cell crisis. (See page 00 for sports in these classifications.)

Sickle cell anemia is found primarily among black people, but it has also been seen in Southern Mediterranean people.

Call the Sickle Cell hotline number (1–800–638–2300) for more information.

These and many other mental and physical illnesses may affect a child's ability to participate fully in strenuous exercise activities. Most often, however, with ongoing medical monitoring, almost every child can enjoy the benefit from some level of sports play. With a clear understanding of your child's capabilities and limitations, you will be able to steer him or her to a specific sport that will enhance the quality of the growing years.

Epilogue

Millions of kids across the country have made sports play the most popular American pastime simply because it's fun, while parents have long recognized and supported athletic programs because they offer valuable lessons in cooperation, competition, sportsmanship, and self-discipline. But despite these positive factors, as a parent you also know that youth athletes often suffer sports-related injuries. That's why young competitors need their parents to do more than drop them off at practices and cheer them on at games. They need them to take an active role in the prevention and care of sports-related injuries. Having read this book, you are obviously an involved parent and are now prepared to keep your young athlete safe from serious injury.

You can use the information from Part I to assure yourself you have a right to stay involved in your child's athletic program. You are not being overprotective when you monitor the use of safety equipment, body conditioning, coaching styles, and team attitudes. You are being a responsible and caring parent.

The sport-specific information in Part II can be kept as a handy resource over the years. As your child experiments with different sports, you'll know what safety factors to look for and what research has found to be the safest and most dangerous aspects of each sport.

The information from Part III will enable you to support and supplement your doctor's involvement in your children's health care. And you can use your knowledge of the ways in which a child's body differs from an adult's to understand why your children need you to supervise, monitor, and nurture their athletic efforts.

This book has been written in the hope of *preventing* future sports-related injuries. While it is quite true that intense physical activity often poses the risk of bodily harm, it is also true that in the realm of athletics, forewarned is truly forearmed.

Appendix A

■ ■ ■ ■

#1

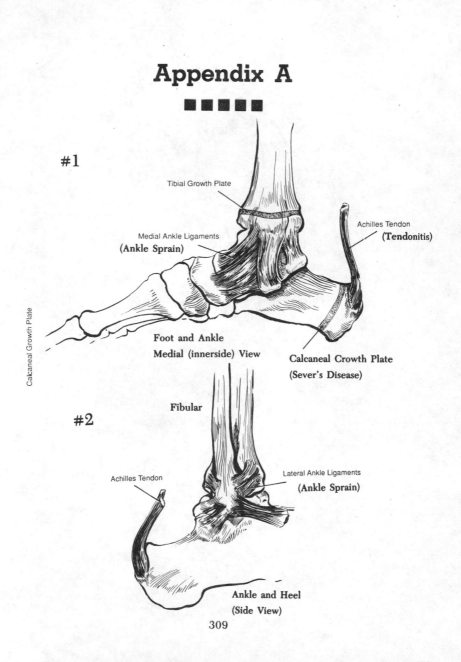

Tibial Growth Plate

Achilles Tendon
(Tendonitis)

Medial Ankle Ligaments
(Ankle Sprain)

Calcaneal Growth Plate

**Foot and Ankle
Medial (innerside) View**

Calcaneal Crowth Plate
(Sever's Disease)

Fibular

#2

Achilles Tendon

Lateral Ankle Ligaments
(Ankle Sprain)

**Ankle and Heel
(Side View)**

#3

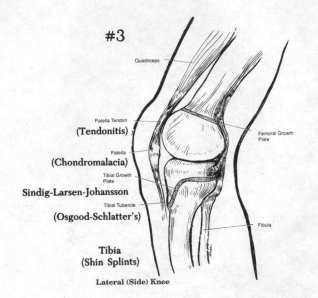

Quadriceps

Patella Tendon
(Tendonitis)

Femoral Growth
Plate

Patella
(Chondromalacia)

Tibial Growth
Plate

Sindig-Larsen-Johansson

Tibial Tubercle

(Osgood-Schlatter's)

Fibula

Tibia
(Shin Splints)

Lateral (Side) Knee

#4

Posterior
Cruciate
Ligament

Anterior Cruciate
Ligament

Medial Collateral
Ligament

Medial
Meniscus

Lateral
Meniscus

Tibial Growth
Plate

Fibula

Anterior (Front) Knee

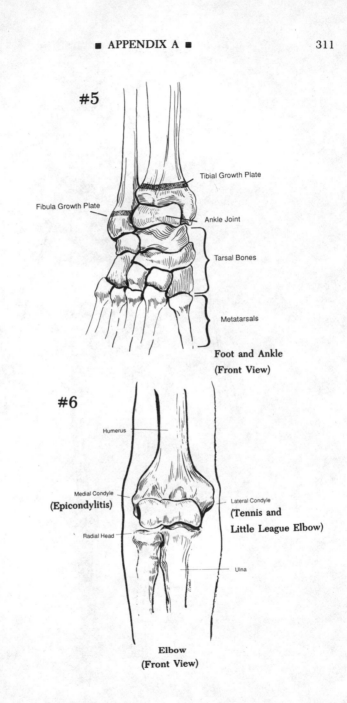

#5

Tibial Growth Plate

Fibula Growth Plate

Ankle Joint

Tarsal Bones

Metatarsals

**Foot and Ankle
(Front View)**

#6

Humerus

Medial Condyle

(Epicondylitis)

Lateral Condyle

**(Tennis and
Little League Elbow)**

Radial Head

Ulna

**Elbow
(Front View)**

#7

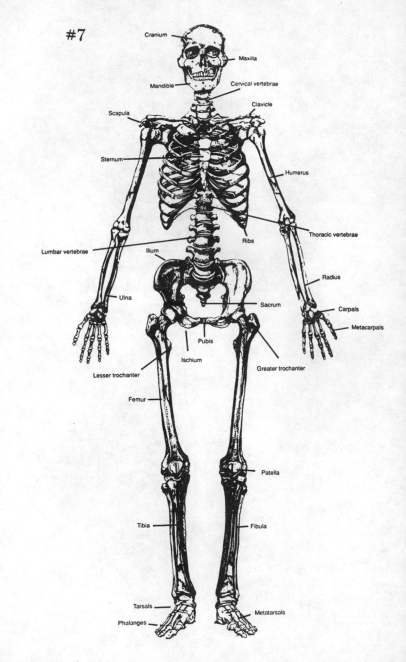

Appendix B

■■■■■

Sports Oganizations

The following organizations have been established to develop, improve, and promote sports participation. They are included in this book to give you a handy resource for further information regarding rules, coaches' training, safety considerations, statistics, league organization, and by-laws. Many also sponsor competitions and offer clinics, films, and educational materials; some publish newsletters and/or magazines. Although some notable sports organizations are not included in this list, it is our belief that the following will have the information you need regarding youth athletics or will be able to refer you to the appropriate source.

Baseball

Little League Baseball
PO Box 3485
Williamsport, PA 17701
717–326–1921

Babe Ruth Baseball
PO Box 5000
1770 Brunswick Ave.
Trenton, NJ 08638
609–695–1434

National Amateur Baseball Federation
12406 Keynote Lane
Bowie, Maryland 20715
301-262-0770

Basketball

National Association of Basketball Coaches of the U.S.
PO Box 307
Branford, CT 06405
203-488-1232

National Wheelchair Basketball Association
110 Seaton Building
University of Kentucky
Lexington, KY 40506
606-257-1623

Football

Pop Warner Football
1315 Walnut Street, Suite 1632
Philadelphia, PA 19107
215-735-1450

For high school information contact:

The National Federation of High School Associations
11724 Plaza Circle Box 20626
Kansas City, Missouri 64195
816-464-5400

Gymnastics

US Gymnastics Federation
Pan Am Plaza
201 S. Capitol Suite 300
Indianapolis, IN 46225
317-237-5050

Ice Hockey

American Hockey Coaches Association
22 Tryon Avenue
Rumford, RI 02916
401–863–1915

Lacrosse

US Women's Lacrosse Association
45 Maple Avenue
Hamilton, NY 13346
315–824–2480

US Lacrosse Coaches' Association (Men's)
University of Delaware
Robert Schillinglaw
302–451–8661

Skiing

U.S. Ski Educational Foundation
PO Box 100
Park City, UT 84060
801–649–9090

Ski For Light (Handicapped skiers)
1455 W. Lake St.
Minneapolis, MN 55408
612–827–3232

Soccer

Soccer Association For Youth
5945 Ridge Avenue
Cincinnati, OH 45213
513–351–7291

Softball

Amateur Softball Association of America
2801 NE 50th Street
Oklahoma City, OK 73111
405-424-5266

National Wheelchair Softball Association
1616 Todd Court
Hastings, MN 55033
612-437-1792

Swimming

National Interscholastic Swimming Coaches of America
Glenbrook South High School
4000 W. Lake Ave
Glenview, IL 60025
708-729-2000

Tennis

US Tennis Association
1212 Avenue of the Americas, 12th floor
New York, NY 10036
212-302-3322

Track and Field

The Athletics Congress/U.S.A.
PO Box 120
Indianapolis, IN 46206
317-638-9155

Achilles Track Club
Nine E. 89th St.
New York, NY 10128
212-967-6496

Volleyball

US Volleyball Association
1750 E. Boulder Street
Colorado Springs, CO 80909
719–632–5551, ext. 3312

Wrestling

USA Wrestling
405 W. Hall of Fame Avenue
Stillwater, OK 74075
405–377–5242

Handicapped Athletes

Special Olympics
1350 New York Ave., N.W., Suite 500
Washington, DC 20005
202–628–3630

Coaches' Education and Certification

American Coaching Effectiveness Program:
This is a group that trains coaches at all levels of sports. It offers instruction through videotapes, books, and clinics. Contact:
ACEP National Center, Box 5076, Champaign, IL 61820
800–747–4457

National Youth Sports Coaches Association
This is a nonprofit organization that was created out of the need to train youth sports coaches. It offers coaching certification to NYSCA members who pledge that the emotional and physical well-being of the children comes before winning. Contact:
NYSCA, 2611 Old Okeechobee Rd, West Palm Beach, FL 33409
407–684–1141

National Association for Sports and Physical Education
This organization is affiliated with the American Alliance for
Health, Physical Education, Recreation and Dance. It is dedicated to improving the total sports and physical education
experience in the United States. It offers competency guidelines for coaches at all levels of competition. Contact:
NASPE, 1900 Association Dr., Reston, VA 22091
703–476–3410

National High School Athletic Coaches Association
This organization offers educational seminars in specific subject areas for coaches and is developing a coaches' certification
program that will require a broad range of courses. Contact:
NHSACA, Box 1808, Ocala, FL 32678
904–622–3660

High School Sports

National Federation of State High School Associations
This organization sells the playing rules that govern virtually
all high school athletic competitions in the United States.
Contact:
NFSHSA, 11724 Plaza Circle, P.O. Box 20626, Kansas City,
MO 64195
816–464–5400

Appendix C

■ ■ ■ ■ ■

Guidelines for Good Coaching

Scientific Bases of Coaching

Medical-Legal Aspects of Coaching

Every young athlete should be provided a safe and healthful environment in which to participate. The coach should have basic knowledge and skills in the prevention of athletic injuries, and basic knowledge of first aid.

Every youth sports coach should:

1. Demonstrate knowledge and skill in the prevention and care of injuries generally associated with participation in athletics.
2. Be able to plan and coordinate procedures for the emergency care of athletes.
3. Be knowledgeable about the legal responsibilities of coaching, including insurance coverage for the coach and athlete.
4. Recognize and insist on safe playing conditions and the proper use of protective equipment.
5. Be able to provide young athletes with basic information

319

about injury prevention, injury reporting, and sources of medical care.

Training and Conditioning of Young Athletes

Every young sport athlete should receive appropriate physical conditioning for sports participation. The coach should use acceptable procedure in their training and conditioning programs.

Every youth sports coach should:

1. Be able to demonstrate the basic knowledge and techniques in the training and conditioning of athletes.
2. Recognize the developmental capabilities of young athletes and adjust training and conditioning programs to meet these capabilities.
3. Know the effects of the environmental conditions (such as heat, cold, humidity, air quality) on young athletes and adjust practice and games accordingly.
4. Be able to recognize the various indications of over-training, which may result in injury and/or staleness in athletes, and be able to modify programs to overcome these consequences.

Psychological Aspects of Coaching

A positive social and emotional environment should be created for young athletes. The coach should recognize and understand the developmental nature of the young athlete's motivation for sport competition and adjust his/her expectations accordingly.

Every youth sports coach should:

1. Subscribe to a philosophy that emphasizes the personal growth of individuals by encouraging and rewarding achievement of personal goals and demonstration of effort, as opposed to overemphasis on winning.

2. Demonstrate appropriate behavior of young athletes by maintaining emotional control and demonstrating respect to athletes, officials and fellow coaches.
3. Demonstrate effective communication skills such as those needed to provide appropriate feedback, use a positive approach, motivate athletes, and demonstrate proper listening skills.
4. Emphasize and encourage discussion of matters concerning the display of sportsmanship in competitive and noncompetitive situations.
5. Be sufficiently familiar with the principles of motivation, including goal setting and reinforcement, in order to apply them in constructive ways.
6. Be able to structure practice and competitive situations to reduce undue stress, and/or to teach young athletes how to reduce any undue stress they experience related to performance.

Growth, Development, and Learning of Young Athletes

Young athletes should have positive learning experiences. The coach should have a knowledge of basic learning principles and consider the influence of developmental level on the athlete's performance.

Every youth sports coach should:

1. Recognize the physical and cognitive changes that occur as children develop and how these changes influence their ability to learn sports skills.
2. Concentrate on the development of fundamental motor and cognitive skills that lead to improvement of specific sports skills.
3. Understand the physical and cognitive differences manifested by early and later maturers.

Techniques of Coaching Young Athletes

Every young athlete should have the opportunity to participate regularly in a sport of his or her choosing. The coach should provide guidance for successful learning and performance of specific sport techniques, based on the maturity level or proficiency of the athlete.

Every youth sports coach should:

1. Know the key elements of sports principles and technical skills and the various teaching styles that can be used to introduce and refine them.
2. Recognize that young athletes learn at different rates and accommodate these differences by flexibility in teaching styles.
3. Be able to organize and conduct practices throughout the season in order to provide maximal learning.
4. Be able to select appropriate skills and drills, and analyze errors in performance.
5. Be able to provide challenging but safe and successful experiences for young athletes by making appropriate modifications during participation.
6. Understand why rules and equipment should be modified for children's sports.

Bibliography

Chapter One

1. Jay Kimiecik, "Who Needs Coaches Education? U.S. Coaches Do," *The Physician and Sportsmedicine*, 16 (November 1988): 124.

Chapter Three

1. American Academy of Pediatrics, *Sports Medicine: Health Care for Young Athletes*, (Evanston, Illinois: American Academy of Pediatrics, 1983), p. 46.
2. American Academy of Pediatrics, *Sports Medicine*, pp. 47–50.
3. National Strength and Conditioning Association, "Position Paper on Prepubescent Strength Training," *National Strength and Conditioning Association*, 7 (November 4, 1985): 29.

Chapter Four

1. Committee on School Health, "School Health Examinations," *Pediatrics*, 67 (1981): 576.
2. American Academy of Pediatrics, *Sports Medicine*, pp. 85–86.
3. Douglas B. McKeag, "Preseason Physical Examination for the Prevention of Sports Injuries," *Sports Medicine*, 2 (1985): 416.
4. American Academy of Pediatrics, *Sports Medicine*, p. 77.
5. R.C. Schineider, J.C. Kennedy, and M.L. Plant, eds., *Sports Injuries Mechanisms, Prevention, and Treatment* (Baltimore: Williams and Wilkins, 1985), p. 621.

6. American Academy of Pediatrics, *Sports Medicine,* pp. 86–88.
7. Schineider, et al., *Sports Injuries,* p. 626.
8. McKeag, "Preseason Physical," p. 427.

Chapter Five

1. Karen Knortz, and Randy Reinhart, "Women's Athletics: The Athletic Trainer's Viewpoint," *Clinics in Sports Medicine,* 3 (October 1984): 852.
2. Elaine Landau, *Why Are They Starving Themselves?* (New York: Julian Messner, 1983), p. 78.
3. W.E. Buckley, C.E. Yesalis and K.K. Friedl, "Estimated Prevalence of Anabolic Steroid Use Among Male High School Seniors," *Journal of the American Medical Association,* 260 (1988): 3441.
4. Janet Nelson, "Why Some Children Opt for Sidelines," *New York Times,* November 6, 1989, p. C12.
5. Bruce Watkins and Amy Montgomery, "Conceptions of Athletic Excellence Among Children and Adolescents," *Child Development,* 60 (December 1989): 1362.
6. F.G. Pillemer and L.J. Micheli, "Psychological Considerations in Youth Sports," *Clinics in Sports Medicine,* 7 (July 1988): 685.

Chapter Eight

1. B. Goldberg, "Injury Patterns in Youth Sports," *The Physician and Sportsmedicine,* 17 (March 1989): 178.
2. Ibid., p. 179.

Chapter Ten

1. J.W. Pritchett, "Cost of High School Soccer Injuries," *American Journal of Sports Medicine,* 9 (1981): 64.
2. D.D. Backous, K.E. Friedl, N.J. Smith, T.J. Parr, and W.D. Carpine, Jr., "Soccer Injuries and Their Relation to Physical

Maturity," *American Journal of Diseases of Children*, 142 (August 1988): 841.
3. U.S. Consumer Product Safety Commission, *Overview of Sports-Related Injuries in Persons 5–14 Years of Age* (Washington, D.C., Dec. 1981).
4. Backous, et al., "Soccer Injuries."

Chapter Thirteen

1. R.K. Requa and J.G. Garrick, "Injuries in Interscholastic Wrestling," *The Physician and Sportsmedicine*, 9 (1981): 44.
2. P.J. Rasch and W. Droll, *What Research Tells the Coach About Wrestling* (Washington, DC,: American Association for Health, Physical Education and Recreation, 1964).

Chapter Fourteen

1. M.F. Rielly, "The Nature and Causes of Hockey Injuries: A Five-year Study," *The Athletic Trainer*, 17 (1982): 88.
2. P.F. Vinger, "Too Great a Risk Spurred Hockey Mask Development," *The Physician and Sportsmedicine*, 5 (1977): 70.
3. F.O. Mueller and C.S. Blyth, "A Survey of 1981 College Lacrosse Injuries," *The Physician and Sportsmedicine*, 10 (1982): 86.
4. C.F. Ettlinger and R.J. Johnson, "The State of the Art in Preventing Equipment-Related Alpine Ski Injuries," *Clinics in Sports Medicine*, 1 (1982): 199.
5. R.J. Johnson, M.H. Pope, and C.F. Ettlinger, "Ski Injuries and Equipment Function," *Journal of Sports Medicine and Physical Fitness*, 2 (1974): 299.

Chapter Fifteen

1. O. Bar-Or, "Importance of Differences Between Children and Adults for Exercise Testing and Exercise Prescription," *Exercise Testing and Exercise Prescription For Special Cases* (Philadelphia: Lea and Febiger, 1987), p. 49.

2. O. Bar-Or, R. Dotan, O. Inbar, A. Rotshtein, and H. Zonder, "Voluntary Hypohydration in 10- to 12-year-old Boys," *Journal of Applied Physiology: Respiratory, Environmental and Exercise Physiology*, 48 (1980): 104.
3. R. Araki, K. Toda, K. Matsuskita, and A. Tsujino, "Age Differences in Sweating During Muscular Exercise," *Japanese Journal of Physical Fitness and Sports Medicine*, 28 (1979): 239.
4. C.J. Hale, "Physiological Maturity of Little League Baseball Players," *Research Quarterly. American Association of Health and Physical Education*, 27 (1956): 276.
5. H.H. Clark, "Characteristics of Young Athletes," *Kinesiology Review* (1968): 33.
6. Kris Berg, "Aerobic Function in Female Athletes," *Clinics in Sports Medicine*, 3 (October 1984): 779.
7. L.F. Tomasi, J.A. Peterson, G.P. Pettit, et al., "Women's Response to Army Training," *The Physician and Sportsmedicine*, 5 (1977): 32.
8. P.A. Whiteside, "Men's and Women's Injuries in Comparable Sports," *The Physician and Sportsmedicine*, 8 (1980) 130.
9. G.J. Erdelyi, "Gynecological Survey of Female Athletes," *Journal of Sports Medicine and Physical Fitness*, 2 (1962): 174.

Chapter Eighteen

1. American Academy of Pediatrics, *Sport Medicine*, p. 104.
2. American Academy of Pediatrics, Committee on Sports Medicine, "Atlantoaxial Instability in Down Syndrome," *Pediatrics*, 74 (1984): 152.
3. S. Livingston, and W. Berman, "Participation of the Epileptic Child in Contact Sports," *Journal of Sports Medicine and Physical Fitness*, 10 (1978): 218.
4. American Academy of Pediatrics, *Sports Medicine*, p. 116.
5. E. Hulse and W.B. Strong, "Preparticipation Evaluation in Athletes," *Pediatric Review*, 9 (1987): 1.
6. American Academy of Pediatrics, *Sports Medicine*, p. 124.